What Do I Say Next? Everyday Mental Health Conversations in Primary Care

A significant problem experienced by some general practitioners (GPs) and many trainees and other primary care health professionals is the challenge of completing a useful and safe consultation with patients with mental health problems within the constraints of a standard-length appointment. These challenges may arise from a lack of specific expertise in this area, poor training in the relevant skills and, perhaps, the attitude that there is not much that the primary care practitioner can do to help.

This new book focuses on enhancing the repertoire of communication skills available for mental health consultations, providing a range of tools and techniques drawn from accepted models, including cognitive behavioural therapy (CBT), transactional analysis (TA), motivational interviewing and acceptance commitment therapy (ACT), illustrating how to apply these within a typical 10–12-minute primary care consultation.

Essential reading for all primary care practitioners in training and practice, the book equips readers with the confidence and knowledge to provide excellent mental health care for their patients.

What Do I Say Next? Everyday Mental Health Conversations in Primary Care

A Practical Guide

Sophie Jadwiga Ball (MBChB, DRCOG, FRNZCGP)

GP and Lead Medical Educator, RNZCGP
New Zealand

Liz Moulton MBE (MBChB, DRCOG, MMEd [distinction], FRCGP)

GP Educator and Freelance GP
UK

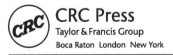

CRC Press
Taylor & Francis Group
Boca Raton London New York

CRC Press is an imprint of the
Taylor & Francis Group, an **informa** business

Designed cover image: Shutterstock 1796499103

First edition published 2025
by CRC Press
2385 NW Executive Center Drive, Suite 320, Boca Raton, FL 33431

and by CRC Press
4 Park Square, Milton Park, Abingdon, Oxon, OX14 4RN

CRC Press is an imprint of Taylor & Francis Group, LLC

ISBN: 9781032529172 (hbk)
ISBN: 9781032513188 (pbk)
ISBN: 9781003409168 (ebk)

DOI: 10.1201/9781003409168

Typeset in Bembo
by Evolution Design and Digital.

Contents

Authors' note

Whilst both authors contributed to the whole book, Liz particularly focused on Section 1 and Sophie on Section 2. The memory tools and mnemonics in this text, such as SEE DEPRESS, "choose the focus" and "vowels of change", were created by Sophie – with many iterations before the final versions. The words *What do I say next?* have frequently been in Sophie's head in her consultations about mental health and addiction.

Acknowledgements

We acknowledge many general practitioners (GPs), nurse practitioners (NPs), nurses, psychologists, psychiatrists, physiotherapists and occupational therapists who work in primary care, mental health and/or addictions. We thank those who reviewed, made contributions and allowed the use of their concepts, as well as those who have taught, guided and inspired us – knowingly or not!

These individuals include Bruce Arroll, Helen Hamer, Karen Fraser, Cassandra Laskey, Brody Runga, Lila O'Farrell, Rob Marchl, David Codyre, Karen Lucas, Rob Shieff, Balveer Sikh, Pam Low, Wayne Hussey, Giresh Kanji, Karen Lucas, Pam Hewlett, Jane Fausett, Tess Ahern, Debra Lampshire, Rudy Bakker, Pete Watson, Clive Bensemann, Jadwiga Ball, Clive Martin, Wendy Brown, Val Williams, Lucy O'Hagan, Brett Mann and others, including all of our trainees, now and in the past.

Authors

Dr Sophie Jadwiga Ball (MBChB, DRCOG, FRNZCGP)

A UK trained GP who has been a passionate educator both in the UK and in New Zealand Aotearoa, where she moved in 2009. She has had various roles with the Royal New Zealand College of General Practice and is currently the Lead Medical Educator for Auckland South. She works clinically at a high-needs practice part-time. She spent seven years as the Primary Care Mental Health and Addictions Clinical Lead for Counties Manukau (South Auckland's District Health Board), leading the design and implementation of a mental health model for primary care, "Wellness Support". This model won Primary Care Mental Health Model of Care in the 2020 inaugural Primary Healthcare Awards, NZ.

Dr Liz Moulton MBE (MBChB, DRCOG, MMEd [distinction], FRCGP)

A GP trainer for 30 years, with a wealth of experience in preparing candidates for the MRCGP, she has also undertaken most roles within Health Education England Yorkshire and the Humber and was Deputy Director of Postgraduate GP Education. She has been a GP advisor to Leeds Health Authority, to the Department of Health and to the RCGP practice support unit. She taught the master's programme for medical education at Leeds University for five years. She currently works as a freelance GP, consultation skills expert and appraiser for GPs and Responsible Officers. She is the author of *The Naked Consultation* and co-author of *The Complete CSA Casebook* and *The Complete MRCGP Casebook*.

Introduction

They are really fidgeting, seem anxious and are avoiding eye contact; they might have low mood. They are looking at me to respond – what do I say next?

We want to share with you what we have learned about how to have useful, manageable mental health conversations within a time-limited primary care consultation.

As primary care clinicians, we frequently encounter people with mental health problems and sometimes rely on a skill set of listening and giving time, medication and referring on to other people. But can we do more? The ideas we present here build on existing skills and are taken from recognised psychological interventions, adapted to be useful in primary care.

If you are already working in primary care, some of these may be approaches you already use but perhaps haven't named or recognised, and others may be new ideas to try out. If you are learning about primary care, then these are some ideas for when you are stuck and ask yourself, *What do I say next?*

Have you experienced any of the following after a mental health consultation?

- Feeling emotionally drained.
- Feeling like you are looking for answers that you don't have.
- Finding you are inevitably running late.

Then this book is for you.

We can relate to all these points. Few of us have been taught how to have a useful, optimistic, time-efficient mental health consultation in a primary

DOI: 10.1201/9781003409168-1

care setting. We might know how to take a history, prescribe or refer, but we may struggle to effectively use consultation time to make a plan that can start as soon as a person leaves the room. In this situation, it is easy to run late and be left dissatisfied and even with a feeling of being burdened. Can we do more than giving time and making onward referrals?

What about the patient? What might their view be of our typical consultation? Some might appreciate us giving our time, listening. They might expect and want medication or referral options. However, some might have other thoughts. We have had our eyes opened, hearing some of these views on the common outcomes of a consultation.

Refer to a psychologist	*Things must be worse than I thought. Even a doctor can't help me. I feel more hopeless. Involving other professionals means waiting, I feel bounced around, and I will have to keep repeating my story.*
A prescription	*I asked for help but all I got was a prescription. I didn't want medication, but there was no other option.*
Lengthy listening	*It was good to talk but what's changed? When I left, everything was still the same.*

Can we make changes to our consultations that benefit our patients and ourselves?

What we could do differently in our consultations

Primary care is busy, and we all consult for most – if not all – of the time without colleagues present. This makes it all too easy to become stuck on the treadmill of consultations, with each following a similar pattern. Using different structures means we have the flexibility to adapt to different people and the approach they need at that time. We can still use our traditional structures and management options and may also choose others, such as holistic, transdiagnostic approaches.

What does this mean? Instead of the conventional "history, diagnosis, management", we think more broadly about the whole person. Transdiagnostic approaches focus on common symptoms that can be present within multiple disorders rather than providing care specific to one disorder or diagnosis. An example is worry. This is a symptom common to many diagnoses. We could focus on defining whether this worry falls more within generalised anxiety disorder or obsessive-compulsive disorder. Or we could consider worry transdiagnostically and aim our discussion and management at the functional impact of the worry.

Holistic approaches are often talked about in health. This moves the focus away from being fixed exclusively on the physical health of an individual. Instead, we consider multiple angles, which include psychological, cognitive, emotional, behavioural and interpersonal aspects. Taking a holistic approach can mean discussing a person's community, religion and the environment. Some cultures, including many indigenous peoples, have always understood health to be defined in this way – as a broader social, emotional, environmental and cultural well-being of the community and its land.

What to expect from this book

The tools we present are practical, realistic ways to include positive and behavioural psychological approaches. They come from evidence-based motivational interviewing, acceptance commitment therapy and cognitive behavioural therapy, adapted for a primary care setting.

We include:

- Simple-to-use questions and short structures that transform an interaction from a list of problems to possible solutions and next steps.
- Specific application of these questions and structures to situations commonly encountered in primary care.
- Demonstrations using scripts of conversations between a health professional and the person attending, based on real situations.

The book is divided into two sections. In Section 1, we cover the parts of the consultation and the theory of the tools. In Section 2, we base the chapters around common presentations in primary care.

What not to expect from this book

We use a transdiagnostic, holistic approach within the tools in this book and so do not describe making diagnoses, medication options and referral pathways. Always use your own clinical judgement.

Sometimes we all wish for a way to make tangible, real changes to someone's situation – their access to money, housing or social opportunity. We wish we could change or delete experiences of violence, injustice or neglect. We are all aware of the need to align social and health sectors and to address wider issues around population health. We do not attempt to discuss these issues. Instead, we share with you some ways to approach your mental health consultations that can create a sense of optimism, positivity and empowerment.

Who is this book written for?

This book is written for anyone working in a primary care or community setting, regardless of role. Depending on your role, some parts of the book will be more relevant than others. We believe that the more primary care team members there are to support mental health, the better, and that nurses, doctors, physicians' associates, pharmacists and others can use these tools.

What about guidelines and research?

We suggest that, to accompany this book, you read and assimilate local mental health pathways and guidelines. We assume that you will complement the tools and techniques in this book with other management. Each person is different and no doubt you will consider all appropriate options, including both medication and non-medication – psychology and other services. As always, make decisions based on a clinical judgement, a person's preferences and evidence-based practice.

When is it appropriate to use these tools?

Context is important. Let's take the common example of someone pre-senting with back pain. Think about how you might approach each of the following:

- A fit and healthy 50-year-old with three days of back pain.
- A 50-year-old with 15 years of back pain and multiple surgeries.

Clearly, there would be differences in gathering information, examining the patient and management, as well as some similarities in these consultations.

Now, let's think about two different presentations of anxiety:

1 A student with an imminent exam experiencing anxiety for the first time.
2 Someone with many years of anxiety preventing them from leaving home.

The tools we will describe can be used in both cases. When symptom duration is short, when there are fewer episodes and/or when there is less impact on function, it is more likely that we would use these tools exclusively. With a longer duration, multiple previous episodes, involvement of other health professionals in the past and/or more impact on function, we would probably use these tools in combination with other management options.

Choice of management will be influenced by a person's preferences and any limitations to the availability and timeliness of local services. As well as using guidelines and our clinical judgement, we seek to be flexible with every person.

Factors such as symptom impact or severity and duration can be used as a guide to management. Sometimes, we use symptom scores alongside our clinical judgement to give us an idea of severity.

Alongside symptoms, we consider complexity. There could be complexity due to the number of medical diagnoses and severity of these, or social complexities such as isolation, housing or employment issues.

The role of the approaches in this book

Figure 1.1 shows how and when we might use the approaches in this book.

GP services refers to primary care and community-based services such as social support agencies, community-based psychology or counselling.

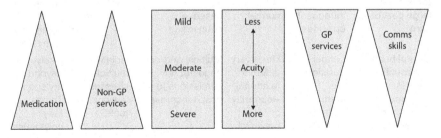

FIGURE 1.1 The role of the approaches in this book.

Non-GP services refers to hospital or secondary care services that may include mental health inpatient services and outpatient psychiatry and psychotherapy.

Medication refers primarily to antidepressants, though it could include medication such as antipsychotics.

Comms (communication) skills means the application of evidence-based psychological tools applied in brief ways by a primary care healthcare provider.

The communication tools and skills described in this book may be used with anyone. We can see from Figure 1.1 that for someone presenting with complex and uncommon symptoms, such as a new psychosis significantly affecting them at home and work, we might use the approaches in this book to discuss a safety plan but would also involve other professionals and discuss medication.

In contrast, for someone who has anxiety but is functioning normally with a good support network of family and friends, we may well use only effective communication skills and the tools in this book.

Factors to consider when deciding the role of the tools in this book

	DURATION/ EPISODES	IMPACT AND SEVERITY	INVOLVEMENT OF OTHER PROFESSIONALS	PERSON FACTORS INCLUDING SUPPORT / SKILLS	SAFETY/ SCOPE
Mental health communication tools are a large part of care	Shorter duration and/or infrequent episodes	Life is quite similar to normal	None or minimal, mainly community based, e.g. counselling	Supportive people, some coping tools	Likely within my scope, seen commonly in my role
Mental health communication tools in combination with other management	Longer duration, e.g. continuous, multiple episodes	Life is very different to normal – currently or previously	Multiple and/or ongoing. Any admissions to hospital or respite	Isolation, multiple stresses, few coping tools	Likely beyond my scope. Things I/my colleagues see less often

A practical example

Annabelle, aged 26.

Presenting problem

I think I have bipolar. In the last few weeks, I have spent a lot of money, I'm drinking too much and I can't sit still. And I am losing weight. I am not sure I can pay the rent this month. My friends say they have had enough of me, but we still hang out. I am safe.

Duration/episodes – short, nil previous

Impact and severity – sounds significant

Involvement of other professionals – none

Person factors including support/skills – financial stress; friends supportive

Safety/scope – possibly a less common presentation

Possible diagnoses – anxiety, hypomania, bipolar disorder, hyperthyroid

The diagnosis and management of a mental health problem such as bipolar disorder is beyond the scope of this book. However, we can still use our holistic primary care approaches to exclude causes such as hyperthyroidism and use transdiagnostic mental health communication tools to work out coping and safety strategies.

Perhaps we talk with Annabelle and find out that she usually copes with support from her partner, but they split up three weeks ago. She has always found shopping comforting, and after the break-up, her friends initially encouraged her to go out and drink. She is now using these strategies more and they are causing problems, such as not eating due to feeling hungover and nauseous. If she doesn't stay busy, her thoughts about her partner become too much, so she is keeping "on the go".

We might explore ways she has coped in the past, prior to the relationship, and make a plan. She told us that she used to follow online make-up tutorials and was in charge of make-up for a local amateur theatre group. While waiting for the blood test results, she will go through her make-up collection and reconnect with one friend still involved with the theatre group. These are manageable next steps.

The layout of this book

We aim to provide a framework for mental health conversations from start to finish. In the first part of the book, we explore the consultation, including:

Section 1

1 **Data gathering** – a structure for information gathering.
2 **Clinical management** – the second half of the consultation including tools such as one-line pivots and brief interventions.
3 **Mental health and the GP curriculum** – learning about mental health.
4 **Models and theory** – the theory that underpins the tools.
5 **Using metaphors** – how metaphors can help.

In the second part of this book, we aim to give you a glimpse into possible future mental health conversations, covering the following common problems and population groups:

Section 2

6 **Anxiety and stress**
7 **Health anxiety**
8 **Low mood and depression**
9 **Young people**
10 **Older adults**
11 **Coping strategies that can cause problems**
12 **Conversations when there is not much time**
13 **Conversations when there is a context of trauma**
14 **Colleagues** – working together and supporting each other

Word for word?

In the past, we have attended educational sessions and felt enthusiastic about models and theories but have been left wondering, *How do I use this in my day-to-day work?* We hope this book answers this. We provide approaches, questions and explanations that can be borrowed and used in primary care conversations. We invite you into our consulting room and encourage you to compare our words with your own, choosing and adapting these approaches so they feel authentic for you and work best for the setting and populations you encounter.

Notes on reading this book

The people you will meet in this guide are amalgamations and generalisations of people we all meet regularly in our work. Any similarity with real people is due to the similarity of human experience.

You will notice that sometimes we provide two questions or comments from the health professional. While these appear to be asked back-to-back, typically we would use the first option and pause, only using the second if needed.

Summary

We hope this book provides an opportunity for you to reflect on what you say in mental health conversations and makes suggestions for alternative options you might not have tried yet.

Through equipping you with new tools, we hope that you will feel positive and empowered when you encounter future patients with mental health issues and will look forward to your consultations with them.

1

Background and framework for mental health consultations

Section introduction

Section 1 offers an overview of the conversation. At the start, we form a partnership with the person and perhaps their family. We may need to consider cultural differences in how we structure the conversations. We can ask, if we are unsure, about pronunciation of names and may share some background information.

In the first part of the conversation, we will mainly gather information as we get to know a person, why they have come and in what context. We suggest tools, such as the mnemonic SEE DEPRESS, as a way to zoom out and cover the main areas of history. We discuss a way to find out more about someone's mental health when they have primarily been talking about their physical health.

Next, we cover management. Here, the focus is on ways to apply brief psychological interventions. These may be used alone or in combination with medication, psychology and referral to specialist services for mental health or social services.

For those who are learning about primary care in the UK, we cover the Royal College of General Practitioners (RCGP) approach to learning and assessing mental health consultations.

We describe the psychological theories that inform the book's conversations and the use of metaphors.

DOI: 10.1201/9781003409168-2

1

Data gathering

The first half of the consultation consists of data gathering, including interpersonal skills such as building rapport.

When people present their story, this rarely starts at the beginning and moves logically through. More often, it is a kaleidoscope of facts, thoughts and emotions, where different pictures tumble in front of us, waiting for us to translate them into our medical frameworks.

There can be a collision of worlds if we impose too much of a health professional framework on the encounter, but there may be confusion if we follow the tumble of information without any structure. Thus, the start of the consultation is a delicate balance of following and leading, clarifying and sharing understanding. In this chapter, we consider skills and tools that can assist with this initial part of a conversation.

Bearing in mind that if consultations go well or go badly, this is likely to be due mainly to what happens in the first half, what skills can we use? What tools will help?

Before we begin

Even before we start a consultation, there are steps we can take to enhance what happens next.

1 The setting – a warm but neutral space, somewhere that feels "safe". For example:
   • Soundproofing from other rooms – it can be off-putting to partially hear conversations from other rooms.

DOI: 10.1201/9781003409168-3

- Neutral decor – what impression do family photos, dying house plants or three days' worth of unwashed coffee cups give?
2 Ourselves – how are we today? How will we "be" in the conversation?
    - How do we dress? What message does this convey?
    - How do we speak? Can we tune in to the patient and speak "with them" rather than at them, communicating as an equal without jargon?
    - How do we demonstrate professionalism?

Beginnings

First impressions count. We convey this in what we say and how we act. At times, this will go smoothly and happen without us consciously thinking about it. However, if someone arrives before we expect, maybe while we are mentally or literally still finishing tasks from a previous consultation, the start may need a conscious effort. We need to be available to start this conversation well, and this may mean taking time to quickly complete a task or set a reminder so we can be fully present and at our best for this conversation.

With people we have not met before, typically introductions will come next – who we are and our role, and who they are. Most of us work with diverse and multicultural populations, and it can be worth learning appropriate ways to address people. Our patients or colleagues may be able to help us with this. We may learn a word or short greeting in the languages of populations we commonly see, as even one familiar word or phrase can increase rapport and help someone relax and feel safe.

There are now evidence-based approaches to use in conversations with different populations that allow respect for cultural protocols and can improve the consultation and its outcomes. To be able to apply these, we may need to clarify a person's cultural identity (the term for this may be ethnicity or race, depending on the common language used where you are located). Then if, for example, we are working with the indigenous Māori population in New Zealand Aotearoa, we would use the Hui process to learn about someone's relationships to land or family and build connections.

Sometimes, starting with an introduction that includes our preferred pronouns and asking a person which pronouns they use may help us gain rapport and create a safe space for the conversation that follows.

Beginning the clinical conversation

The start of the clinical conversation is one of the most important times in the consultation – the golden minute. Sometimes we might not need any words, only to confirm we have the person we expect in the room. We give attentive non-verbal indicators, with eye contact and turning our body away from a computer and towards the person.

Other times we may use a warm but neutral opening,

How can I help you today?

If said with warmth, genuine interest and a smile, this can help us get off to a good start. In a face-to-face consultation, we may choose to start with,

What brings you in today?

This has the advantage of removing any inferred power imbalance, that is, giving the impression of *I need to help you because you are unable to help yourself.*

Less good starts may crowd the person's thoughts,

I can see you came in just recently with ear problems and mentioned hip pain. Have you had the X-ray yet? Is that why you are here today?

What is wrong with this? As they sit down, the person almost certainly has their brain filled with things they want to say: thoughts, symptoms, worries, hopes about what you, the clinician, might do, things they mustn't forget to include and what their spouse/partner thinks. Asking a closed or semi-closed question means that the person needs to come out of their "story" and consider the question you have asked.

Open questions – ones that can't be answered with yes/no or a short factual answer

When someone comes to a natural pause in their narrative flow, the most efficient and useful thing we can do is encourage them to continue their story. We may use silence and non-verbal cues – eye contact, smiling and nodding – or use one of these approaches:

- Repeat their last two or three words, pause and maintain eye contact.
- Ask a specific but open question or a statement used as a question,

    Can you tell me how that feels?

I'm interested to hear more about X.

- A really good question to get a sense of time frames is,

  How did it start?

This is a much higher-yield question than *When did it start?* – though this is, of course, important to know.

If my calf pain or depression started 10 years ago, a month ago or yesterday, it makes a big difference to the possible differential diagnosis and management. Knowing "how long" is important, but asking **how** it started will almost certainly give you the answer to **when**, as well as a lot more detail. It is also an open question, encouraging the patient to open up and tell you more, whereas,

When did it start? is a closed question, meaning the person may stop relaying their narrative.

In contrast,

How did it start? is an open, high-yield question.

Reminder – closed, semi-closed and open questions

A **closed** question is one that can be answered with "yes" or "no" or with a similar, very specific, binary answer:

- *Did this start last week?* – answer "yes" or "no".
- *Which arm hurts?* – answer "right" or "left".

A **semi-closed question** is one that can only be answered with a fairly limited range of answers:

- *When did it start?* – answer Tuesday, a week ago, last month, many years ago.
- *Did your arm ache, or was it a sharp pain or burning pain or throbbing?* – answer one of the above limited range of options.

An **open question** is one that **can't** be answered yes or no or from a limited range of prescribed options:

- *How did it start?* – answer is likely to be a description.
- *How did your arm feel?* – again, likely to be a description of symptoms that the person experienced.

Open and closed questions – exceptions

There are a few occasions when we may learn more by asking closed questions:

1 Young people may be nonplussed by open questions and may struggle to answer. If we have tried a few open questions and got nowhere, it may be worth asking easy closed questions simply to start to get the young person to start talking.

2 When others, as well as young people, are struggling with open questions, we can try a closed then an open question.

   Closed – *Are things better today than last week or worse?*

   Open – *Tell me in what ways things are better/worse.*

This may get the conversation going.

Closed questions (ones where the answer is short and factual and may be yes/no)

If open questions give us the richest yield of information, why do we need closed questions? Few people tell us everything that we need to know – they probably don't know the risk factors, red flags or significance of family history. There are important pieces of information that we need to find out, and a series of questions that can be answered yes/no or similar is an important adjunct to the narrative. After we have learnt everything we can from active listening, we ask questions to fill in any gaps. These are often short questions that can be answered yes/no or with a brief answer.

Why don't we ask closed questions earlier in the consultation, perhaps to clarify a detail? A common pitfall is to try to clarify a specific detail early on. The problem with this is that once the patient starts answering questions with short answers, their narrative may dry up whilst they wait for us to ask the next question. This then becomes time-inefficient, and it will take us longer to find out everything we need to know, working through an extensive number of closed questions.

Identifying a mental health component

People may present with an overt mental health issue,

I'm feeling depressed.

... or tell us that they want to talk about physical and mental health issues,

I've got this pain in my stomach, and I need to sort out my mental health.

... or the issues may be intertwined and combine physical, mental, social and cultural issues,

I'm so worried about these stomach aches that I can't eat or sleep. I am caring for my dad, who is now terminally ill. I need to prioritise him and have had to stop working.

If someone makes a statement including a mental health diagnosis, like in the first example,

I'm feeling depressed.

... we should not be tempted to assume we know what this means. We may perhaps interpret this as feeling low, having poor concentration and motivation, and being unable to sleep. However, the person may be experiencing a completely different set of symptoms and behaviours – snapping at their children, putting off important work, being angry and not socialising.

At other times, there may be no verbal mention of a mental health issue, but one may be communicated non-verbally; someone might be talking quietly, with minimal responses, looking on the brink of tears. We may then need to open the conversation,

How is your mood?

... or do so more specifically, reflecting the patient's verbal and non-verbal communication,

You said things are fine – and I might be wrong – but the way you are sitting leaning forward, with your arms wrapped around yourself, and talking quietly, makes me wonder if, underneath that feeling fine, there are some other emotions?

Cues

Cues are the clues in the consultation, the hyperlinks or shortcuts that may efficiently take us to what someone is really concerned about. We sometimes hear, *I haven't got time to pick up cues* – but this misses the point. We haven't got time to **miss** cues, particularly in a mental health consultation.

Cues take many forms, but we can learn to spot them with practice. Watching and listening to our recorded consultations will help. Typically, cues are words, phrases or non-verbal clues that stand out from the patient's story. For example:

- A person is mentioned – who are they? Why mention them? What do they think?
- Work is mentioned – how is this relevant?
- An emotionally laden word or phrase is used (*awful, the worst ever, really down*).
- There is a mismatch between words and looks – the patient says something really sad but is laughing.
- Anything that is said twice – on the second occasion, pick it up and explore the cue.

And some cues, like the person looking sad, may be elephants in the room – difficult subject matter we are all skirting around, such as a mental health issue. If there is an elephant, name it and bring it into the conversation. Remember, the larger the "elephant", the more space it will need. So the earlier we identify it, the better; address it either now or in a planned future conversation.

Common themes

In the first part of any consultation, regardless of whether the presentation is a physical issue, mental health issue or a combination, there will be information we want to find out:

- The nature, duration and impact of the presenting issue or symptom.
- Why has the person come with this problem today?
- What are their priorities and expectations?
- The psychosocial context – who is this person in the context of their life?
- What are their thoughts and worries about what is going on.
- How is the problem affecting the person? How is this person's behaviour or action/inaction making the problem better or worse?
- Are they safe?

Finding out more about the symptoms

The key elements that we need to know about are:

- Duration – how long?
- Impact – how is it affecting someone?
- Severity – how bad has it been?

These are all questions to ask at appropriate moments – as part of the conversation and flowing logically and naturally from what has been said by the patient so that there is fluency, like in a conversation with your friend.

Finding out more about the person

In all consultations, whether for physical or mental health, it is as important to find out about the person as it is to find out about their symptoms, problems or worries. Perhaps particularly in mental health conversations, we also want to find out who is in their "team", as this will be relevant to our clinical management.

How do we find out about this person?

- There may be clues in the narrative ("my partner", "at work", "in my running club").
- There may be information in the notes.
- We can ask, using an interested tone of voice and maintaining eye contact,

    We haven't met before – I'm interested to know more about you.
    Tell me who's at home.
    How about work – what do you do? Tell me more about that.

To find out about the team around the person, we might ask,

Who are the people around you that you can talk to?

How do you get on with colleagues at work?

Are there others, perhaps people you haven't contacted for a while?

We might ask about other connections with people:

- Family, friends, people you see regularly.
- Community links – sports groups, religious groups, community groups.
- Healthcare providers, including counselling, workplace support and complementary medicine providers.

And, perhaps later, we might ask,

If we were to include someone as a safety backup, who might that person be?

Finding out about what someone is thinking, worrying about and hoping we might do

ICE is a useful acronym to remind us to ask the questions in this triad, but the words "ideas, concerns, expectations" are not words we naturally use in conversation and can sound formulaic. These questions are not optional, or "nice to know when we remember", but are essential questions. The answers to these will enrich our picture of what is going on for someone and can form an incredibly useful part of a summary before we move into clinical management. We might ask,

What thoughts have you had about all of this?

What's gone through your mind?

What's worried you about …?

In the middle of the night, what's your worst fear about …?

And, generally, later in the consultation,

I already have some thoughts about what we could do, but what thoughts did you have about what might happen next?

Being time-efficient

In primary care, we are usually time-limited, and need to use our time wisely. We must be efficient. What are our efficiency tools?

- Focused open questions – ones that enable the person to talk but nudge them towards what we need to hear, for example,

    Tell me more – may be too vague.

    Tell me more about how this has affected you in the last week – might be a better question because it is both open and focused.

- Closed questions – for specifics such as risk factors and red flags so that we tie up any loose ends before we move into clinical management.

- Curiosity – remember this is not a soap opera, and we don't have all day. We could have a very long and absolutely fascinating conversation with some of the people we see, but we need to pay attention to what's important today and avoid going down rabbit holes. For example, we may really be interested in why their partner left, but this may have limited relevance to this person's priorities for this conversation.

Positive psychology in action

We can use positive psychology in our data gathering to start to nudge the person forward, even before we get to clinical management. Rather than getting into a mutual spiral of *Isn't it awful… I know… I know…*, we can pair empathetic reflections with positively phrased nudge questions:

Reflection – *Life has been really difficult these last few months.*

Nudge question – *What have you managed to keep doing at the most difficult times?*

… or paired reflections/nudge reflections:

Reflection – *Things are really tough for you right now.*

Nudge reflection – *Even though things are really tough, you have managed to keep going with all the things you need to do.*

Key points to cover in mental health data gathering

There are many aspects to a mental health consultation. The mnemonic SEE DEPRESS may help us to remember the key points. Of course, these questions and answers can occur in any order and should be conversational so that there is a logical flow.

S – See the impact – *Since feeling like this, can you see a difference in anything you are doing, or not doing, in daily life compared with before this? How about with your sleep/eating/work/time outside of work? Do you think anyone else has noticed? Has anyone commented on this?*

E – Exacerbating – *Did something happen that seemed to trigger/ worsen how you are feeling?*

E – End point – *Will this reach a conclusion/Is there a date this has to be completed?*

D – Duration – *How long have you been feeling like this?*

E – Episodes – *Have there been times in the past when you have felt similarly to this or when you have noticed your mental health not being good in other ways?*

P – People – *Who is supporting you at the moment?*

R – Risky behaviour and risk factors – *Are you drinking alcohol or using non-prescribed drugs? Recent changes – Any recent life events such as job loss, redundancy, separation or divorce?*

E – Experiment – *What have you tried so far? How did you find that?*

S – Safety – *When things have felt at their worst, what thoughts have you had? Have things got so bad that you have thought of ending your life? Do you have any concerns about your safety at home? Is there any-one who makes you feel unsafe?*

S – Setting – What's the background? Consider important influenc-ing factors such as family history, adverse childhood events (ACEs), trauma, abuse, chronic conditions or head injuries. *Do you think there are things that have happened in the past that might be affect-ing how your health is now?*

Useful tools in data gathering in mental health conversations

We have recognised that there is a mental health aspect to a presentation. Now, we need to explore some specific areas during data gathering. This section outlines some tools that will help us with this task:

*   Coping questions.
*   Treasure hunt.
*   Detective, judge, court reporter – identify, assign, discuss.
*   ABC.
*   Safety and suicide questions.

Coping questions

Identifying current coping strategies is a core element of a mental health conversation, and we will make use of these strategies in our management.

Whenever someone is describing their problems or distress in a way that makes us think that these are having a significant impact, we need to find out their current strengths and strategies. Remember, the person in front of us has probably had their symptoms for some time before coming in to have this conversation. If we can understand the parts of life that have not been affected and how they are managing to keep doing these, we find out current coping strategies. We want to learn more about what is helping them cope so that we can build on any strengths and strategies in our clinical management.

We could ask,

> How are you coping?

But this is unlikely to give us tools, strategies or strengths and may well be answered with, *Badly* or *I'm not*, which does not move the conversation forward.

Instead, we want to phrase the question to specifically find out strengths and not "how" but "what",

> With all the things that have been happening that you were talking about just now, what are the ways you have been coping?

This question includes the phrase, *you have been coping,* and asks **what** the person has done that has helped.

Choosing coping questions

Other questions we could use might be,

How have you been coping with all this going on?

How have you kept your head up through this?

What's kept you afloat while this has all been happening?

What are the things that have been helping you manage at the moment?

What do you do that makes things more bearable?

What's been getting you through?

We can experiment with a couple of questions and find the ones that feel authentic for us to use in our mental health conversations.

Treasure hunt

The treasure hunt principle is that we are looking for something that is missing (the metaphorical treasure) that would improve life if added back. We hunt for it by asking questions to find out what is different with life now compared with a point in the past when things felt differently. We might ask someone, after they tell us they have had depression for a year or so,

What has life been like, overall, the last 12 months, with feeling this depression?

After hearing the answer to this general overview question, we can ask a more time-defined question, asking about the more immediate impact.

In what ways has life been different in the last month, compared with before?

Someone may answer that, a year ago, they were an avid football fan, never missing a game. Now that they have lost their job, they can't afford a season pass and feel disconnected from other fans. Knowing this may allow us to explore if this is still an interest and open a conversation about ways to connect with others and restart watching matches, even if they are unable to be present at the stadium.

Detective, judge and court reporter – identify, assign, discuss

We use this tool to explore the presenting symptoms, uncovering other aspects. Typically, in primary care, people first describe a physical symptom, but this may have other facets related to mental health or social or cultural issues.

We start by using treasure hunt questions to explore the situation and what is different now compared with before. This is the "detective hat". Next, we try and understand which symptoms may be responsible for any areas of distress, the "judge hat". Once we have a theory, we share this and discuss with a person how accurate they think this may be, the final "court reporter hat".

Typically, we would use this with mental and physical health, but it could be that the different elements are mental health and family or culture. Here is an example of a summary connecting mental health, family and culture,

You have mentioned that you are feeling depressed and missing your grandmother. You were close to her but couldn't see her before she died or attend the funeral. You notice your mood is worse around the time of the anniversary of her death. The main problem for you now is struggling with getting things done, perhaps due to your mental health, and things are worse around the anniversary. You said that culturally it is important for you to find a way to say goodbye to your grandmother, and I wonder if addressing this might help your overall well-being. What do you think?

ABC

This tool, often used in psychology, explores a specific event. We can structure our questioning about this event to find out what happened before, what happened at that time and what happened next. Asking these questions enables us to stay curious, open and non-judgemental. The origins of the approach come from behavioural psychology, which explores the links between environments and behaviours:

- **A** – Antecedents – "before"
- **B** – Behaviours – "actions"
- **C** – Consequences – "next"

In the example of someone who binge eats when stressed, we might ask about a recent episode.

Antecedents

Before you started bingeing,

What triggered this?

What were you thinking?

What were you feeling?

What else did you do?

Was there a final trigger that "tipped" you to do this?

To find out different facets (thinking/feeling/doing), it is generally better to ask separate questions. If we ask an amalgamated question, we will rarely hear the answer to all three aspects, instead probably getting the answer to only one.

Sometimes, however, we may ask an amalgamated question to enable someone to give us the easiest and uppermost response before they tackle other "harder" aspects,

What were you thinking or feeling?

Behaviour

We phrase these questions to be non-judgementally curious – exploring in a neutral way without blaming or criticising, simply finding out,

When you were deciding to start eating, did you think about doing anything else?

At that moment, what outcome were you hoping for?

Consequences

What happened straight away after you started eating?

What were you thinking and feeling at that moment?

What did you do?

How did others respond?

How do you feel now looking back?

We conclude with a summary. This allows someone to clarify, add or correct anything we have got wrong. Hearing this summary can be very powerful in its own right, leading to insights or ideas of how to approach the same situation in future.

Safety and suicide questions

We want to check for risks to safety that might come from others or from the person themselves. Asking about suicide does not increase the risk of this happening, and often people are relieved to be able to discuss this.

These are important questions, but they can be hard for us to ask or hard to ask in an effective way. For example, if we were to ask,

You haven't had any thoughts about hurting yourself, have you?

... this would be a closed negative question, which invites the answer "no" or "of course not", so we could all move on – phew. However, even if someone had thoughts of self-harm or suicide and was willing to talk about these, it would be difficult for them to answer "yes" if the question were phrased in this way. How can we start to explore thoughts of suicide?

We can ask a general question and follow this with a specific question if needed.

General question

When things have felt at their worst, what thoughts have you had?

This question may or may not be answered with thoughts about suicide. This may be because the person has no thoughts of self-harm, because they are unsure about how to tell us or because they are apprehensive about how we might react. Will we panic or tell someone? Will we send them to hospital or call the police?

If we are unsure about an answer, we normalise these thoughts and ask a more precise question.

Precise question

It is very common in these situations to have thoughts like it would be better off falling asleep and not waking up; what thoughts have you had like this?

Here we have normalised the thinking – *it is very common in these situations* – and asked an open question, that is,

What thoughts have you had like this? – open

... rather than,

Have you had thoughts like this? – closed – yes/no

If someone tells us they have had these thoughts, either in response to these questions or by volunteering a passing comment, we need to explore this. It is important for us to be alert to cues around suicide – *Things are worse than ever* or *I don't know how I can carry on* – and ask,

When things have been difficult, what thoughts have gone through your head?

Have there been any times when you have worried about staying safe?

If we think there is a risk, but someone will not talk about it or stops mid-way through a conversation, or if answers do not seem congruent, we may want to explore the context of the conversation. We may even consider if there is someone else in the practice whom the person might prefer to talk to and who might be available to have this conversation now,

You mentioned having thoughts about ending your life. I understand this is difficult to talk about. What puts you off talking further about this at the moment? Is there someone else you might prefer to talk to?

Or we may need to make a comment around safety and the limits of confidentiality,

It is hard for me to know how safe you are without us talking further, and to keep you safe, if I am unsure, I will need to involve other people. Can we talk about who might be involved? Or would it be OK to talk a little more about your safety?

It is common for people to have passive thoughts of suicide, such as *I hope I don't wake up; I can't face another day like this.* This can lead to important conversations about strategies for the situation or perception of it. It is less common and more concerning if these thoughts form a plan, with actions decided, or if the thoughts are persistent and intrusive, causing distress.

Detecting those who will successfully commit suicide is immensely challenging. Screening questionnaires such as the Patient Health Questionnaire-9 (PHQ-9) depression screen includes a suicide question, and the Suicide Assessment Five-Step Evaluation and Triage (SAFE-T) questionnaire offers a five-question approach. The sensitivity and specificity of screening tools vary, but none is 100% accurate and we must consider the person and the whole clinical picture. Important factors to remember include:

- Previous or recent self-harm.
- Family history of suicide.
- High risk groups, e.g. over 65 years and 14–24 years.
- Risk factors such as major depression, bipolar or substance use.
- Access to means, including medication.

The tools TPA and HOLLA 321 are a way to start discussions about suicide risk and safety. Additionally, SEE DEPRESS covers areas relevant to suicide screening. The "R" includes recent changes. This could identify activities that are associated with suicidal intent, for example someone getting their affairs in order, seeing people they haven't seen in a long time or having purchased a weapon. The "P" includes the important protective factor of interpersonal relationships, including family, friends and dependent children. All this information will help form an overall clinical impression of the current risk and help you decide on the appropriate next steps.

Discussing safety – thoughts, plans and actions (TPA)

Here is a way to remember suicide questions based around thoughts, plans and actions (TPA).

These questions focus on what has happened or is happening now (past and present).

Thoughts   *When things have felt at their worst, what **thoughts** have you had? Have things got so bad that you have **thought** of ending your life?*

Plan   *Have you thought about – or decided on – a particular **plan** for how you would end your life? In the past, have you had a **plan**?*

Action   *Have you taken any steps towards putting this into **action**? Have you decided what the first step would be? Have you **taken action** in the past?*

Any positive responses to plan and/or action questions would need to be fully explored with careful consideration of current safety and immediate involvement of a wider team.

Commonly, someone may reveal thoughts with no plan or actions. In this case, we would continue with the HOLLA questions.

Discussing safety – HOLLA 321

If someone tells us about thoughts of suicide, but we are reassured there is no plan or action, we can use three HOLLA questions to explore the current situation and ways to stay safe in the future.

How Often? *How often do you find yourself having these types of thoughts of wishing you didn't wake up?*

Long-Lasting? *Do the thoughts come into your head and go again quickly, or do they stick around?*

Act *Do they bother you? Do you think you would ever act on these? What would you do if these thoughts were making you want to act? In that situation, what would keep you safe?*

If these questions bring up uncertainty about safety, we will carefully consider the need to involve a wider team. If we have little or no concern, then Chapter 12 provides some strategies and next steps for a primary care plan for safety using HOLLA as a starting point.

Towards the end of data gathering

As we prepare to start a conversation about clinical management, we should mentally check that we have found out everything we need to know, for example:

- Duration/impact/severity.
- Psychosocial – home, work, what matters to the person, the "team" – we could verbally summarise this.
- Thoughts, worries, what the person hopes you might do (ideas, concerns and expectations).
- Safety issues.

If anything is missing, ask it now.

Summary

Take time to think about the best ways to start conversations because starting well can make a big difference to the whole conversation. Consider learning more about creating a safe space for different populations, considering age, ethnicity, gender or sexuality. We need to be flexible to meet the needs of different groups.

General communication skills such as open questions and asking about ideas, concerns and expectations are, of course, relevant in mental health conversations and can be complemented by specific questions or tools.

We suggest introducing the idea of mental health early in a conversation rather than discussing only a physical problem and then having insufficient time left to discuss a mental health problem.

The mnemonic SEE DEPRESS may remind us of the important areas of data gathering for mental health. Considering safety is paramount, and TPA and HOLLA 321 can provide a structure for discussing suicide and the risk of self-harm.

2

Clinical management: the second part of the consultation, including interpersonal skills

In this chapter, we consider general approaches to clinical management and a broad overview of the second half of the consultation – how we know that we have got to the end of data gathering and what we need to do now. We describe the structures that underpin safe and effective clinical management. In Section 2, we will consider specific management tools to help patients in particular situations or with a particular problem.

Sometimes, experienced clinicians appear to blend data gathering and clinical management so that they listen to something the patient says, offer a suggestion, then ask more questions and modify that suggestion, and so on. For those who are less experienced, and particularly with clinical consultation skills exams, including the MRCGP in mind, it is better to clearly separate the two halves of the consultation as far as possible so that we have enough information before we signal a clear move to clinical management. In general, we should not be asking many data-gathering questions in this part of the consultation.

What do we need to do in the second half of the consultation?

The tasks we complete in clinical management will depend on our role. We may offer an assessment of the problems; make and state an impression

DOI: 10.1201/9781003409168-4

or diagnosis; discuss investigations, prescriptions or referrals; and nego-tiate a plan. It is vital that this continues to be a conversation, that is, a dialogue, and not a monologue in which we are talking "at" the person rather than with them.

When do we know that the first half of the consultation is finished?

There is always more that could be said and more that we could explore about the person's problems, but within a time-limited primary care consultation, we need to decide when we know enough to move on. We need to manage our time well and efficiently so that we do not spend the entire duration of the consultation on data gathering. We will know that we have reached this point when:

- We have a good idea of why the patient has come today.
- We have asked or heard and explored the patient's own thoughts, worries and expectations.
- We have noticed and responded to any cues – verbal and non-verbal.
- We know what the patient might have in mind about what we could do for them today – whether or not this is reasonable or appropriate.
- We know enough about the person in the context of their life – who is at home and how things are.
- We have explored current coping strategies and who is in their team, and who, or what, is pulling in the opposite direction.
- We have found out about the impact – how the problem is affecting the person and whether or how much it is interfering with their life.
- We have asked about and explored risk factors – e.g. alcohol use, family history of depression and previous history of mental health issues of any sort.
- We have checked for red flags and considered self-harm or suicide risk.

How do we move from data gathering to clinical management?

We can signal a transition to the second part of the consultation with a summary of key points,

You have felt anxious for around six weeks now, since the promotion at work. You have had similar episodes in the past, usually getting through these yourself but once seeing a private counsellor. The anxiety is making you delay decisions, and your boss has commented on this. You are trying to work from home when you can, which seems to reduce your anxiety. Your partner is a big support, but is out during the day. Walking together at the end of the day helps you de-stress before bed.

Perhaps we could talk a bit more about feeling anxious and see if there are other options or strategies that you might want to try?

To diagnose or not?

An initial step in clinical management is typically to suggest a diagnosis. If we see someone with Bell's palsy or carpal tunnel syndrome, we generally wouldn't hesitate to name a specific diagnosis. In contrast, in a mental health conversation, sometimes we may miss out the step of stating an impression or differential diagnosis and go straight from data gathering to a clinician-centred approach to clinical management,

OK – my thoughts are that we should…. What do you think?

Why might this be? We may find it hard to put a name to a mental health problem; the "diagnosis" may not be clear cut. There can be big implications to these types of diagnoses with consequences for future careers, health insurance and other areas of life. We might hesitate because of fear of causing upset or experiencing emotion in response to a mental health label.

On other occasions, a person may have come in and opened with, *I think I'm depressed*, and, having talked to them and completed data gathering, we find that we agree and may move into management without explicitly confirming that we are all on the same page with the diagnosis.

If we are using a transdiagnostic approach, we are not seeking to make a diagnosis but rather to identify a core process that underpins a broad range of presentations – and this is the approach we take in this book.

Introducing a diagnosis

Sometimes, it will be useful to discuss a diagnosis or differential, and some exams and assessments, such as the RCGP's simulated consultation assessment, will require this step. We will generally have asked a person's thoughts during data gathering, but, if we have forgotten it, we can ask this now. When we state an impression, diagnosis or differential, it is important to include and incorporate what the person has told us about **their** ideas,

> *You thought you might be depressed. From what you have told me, with your low mood, poor sleep and appetite, and trouble getting going with things – I agree.*

Or

> *You thought you might be depressed – after listening to what you've said, I'm not so sure. It seems to me that the overriding issue is probably anxiety rather than depression. What do you think? Does that sound possible to you?*

We might want to use a transdiagnostic approach, saying,

> *You mentioned that you thought you might be depressed. Whether or not you meet the clinical criteria for depression, it sounds to me that the biggest difference you are noticing is that your world has shrunk down due to not feeling motivated to do many of the things you used to do. I wonder if it is worth us focusing on how we can expand life again. What do you think?*

Sometimes, we can't actually make a diagnosis but can reflect on the main issues causing distress. A university student has come in tearful, though not depressed, feeling overwhelmed with trying to complete coursework and find time for a part-time job to support herself financially. She is clearly distressed and struggling, though no specific diagnosis fits, so we might reflect,

> *I'm hearing that things have been difficult and you are struggling with motivation. Some of the important things to you right now are progressing with your course and working part-time because that is how you pay your rent. How does that sound? Are we on the right track, or perhaps other things feel more important right now?*

If, in response, a person agrees with a verbal "yes" that is congruent with non-verbal body language such as nodding, gestures and eye contact, then we are in agreement. If we think there might be uncertainty in the tone of the "yes" or from non-verbal communication, it is worth responding to this mismatch at this point in the consultation. Noticing and discussing any difference in opinion now will be more helpful than ignoring and continuing with management. In general, people will avoid conflict, and we will need to be open verbally and non-verbally to allow this conversation. Use of the third person can help. We might ask,

> *Do you think your partner/work colleagues/family would agree or disagree with this? Why do you think that? Does that match with what you think?*

> *I have not been living with this as you have, but, from our conversation so far, I think this is likely. I am interested to know what else you think could be going on if this is not correct?*

How can we have a shared approach to management and discuss this with the patient?

A shared approach to management is important in all consultations, but perhaps particularly so when there are mental health issues. If someone has hypothyroidism, then prescribing thyroxine is likely to be the most important thing that we can do today and it is very likely that this medication will help that person to start to feel better and get back on track.

It is a different situation with mental health problems – there is rarely one solution that will, in isolation, make someone feel better. There are always other strategies that we need to use as well, and we can usefully classify these into three groups:

1 Things the patient can do.
2 Things others can help us with.
3 Things we, as health professionals, can do.

Remembering this trio will help us formulate a holistic plan and ensure that we don't miss an important strategy. We will consider each of these three areas of strategy further, using an example, and then expand on the clinical management tasks that the heath professional may complete.

Example

Janet is 38 and calls to tell us that she feels depressed again and has restarted her antidepressants but doesn't have many left. She asks if she can have some more and says that she feels like "a failure". Her mood is low, she lacks motivation and, at times, it is hard to get up and dressed and leave the house. She works in a call centre where management is "on her back" because she is slower than others, and she has had a warning. She needs her job for the income and definitely doesn't want time off.

She had one previous episode of depression last year when she stopped the antidepressants after two months because she was better and didn't need them. In data gathering and through asking specific questions, some of the other information we know is:

- Alcohol – *I've cut right down now.*
- Movement – *I thought about joining a gym to increase exercise, but I'm not sure I would use the membership and the cost of this is a worry.*
- Sleep – *I have trouble getting off to sleep and lie awake worrying. Then, I will go on my phone and check social media to try and relax.*

What can the person do?

Janet has already reduced her alcohol, thought about increasing exercise and tried out using social media to relax.

You ask Janet what she might add in as a next step to support her physical and mental health. Strategies that Janet may suggest could include:

- Lifestyle measures such as eating more fruit and vegetables and less processed food and moving more.
- Following sleep hygiene strategies to improve sleep.
- Cutting down or stopping alcohol or other drugs.
- Taking time to do things that help and doing less of things that have been found to be unhelpful or aggravated the problem. For example, meeting a particular friend is always a supportive and positive experience, but meeting a different one has a more negative impact.
- Taking up or rekindling interests or hobbies, particularly if they involve movement or being with others, for example a sports group or community choir.
- Practising strategies that have been learned previously, cognitive behavioural therapy (CBT) techniques or breathing exercises.

What can others help us with?

Others might include professionals, such as those from social services, health coaches, counsellors, psychologists or psychiatrists. They may also include supportive friends and family or work colleagues. Peer support means involving people with lived experience to support a person.

In data gathering, we have asked about people involved in the person's life – their team – now we can discuss who else might be useful to involve and in which areas, e.g. Janet might have a friend to go walking with and her sister to phone if feeling down late at night. We may also see if we can help grow the team by encouraging the person to identify others who are perhaps currently more peripheral, e.g. speaking to her boss about her health.

What can the health professional do?

We could simply issue the further prescription she has requested, but there are many more useful strands that we can use instead or in addition. We consider here first using the E-tools below, and then other tasks the health professional may complete.

Useful E's[1]

Think of all the Es we can use when talking to Janet:

1 Explain
2 Encourage
3 Educate
4 Empower
5 Elephants

We can **explain** about depression – *it is not uncommon for depression to recur and you are not "a failure" because this has happened.*

We can **encourage** – *this will get better and there are lots of things that can help.*

We can **educate** – *most people need to take antidepressants for longer than two months. After a couple of months, many people start to feel better and therefore stop – but it is common for this improvement not to be sustained. This time, you may want to consider taking the tablets for longer, and we can decide together when and how to stop them.*

We can **educate** about alcohol and **encourage**,

> *It's great that you've cut alcohol right down – that's a really positive step for your health. And we know that alcohol is a depressant drug – it may make you feel relaxed and take the edge off symptoms when you take it, but*

it interferes with sleep and depresses mood. If you can cut down even further and, ideally, stop, that would be a really positive move for your mental health and could help you to start feeling better more quickly.

We can **educate** and **empower** about exercise,

You were thinking about the gym but worried about committing to a membership and then not using it – and it being a drain on your family finances, which are strained.

But it's really good that you were thinking about exercise because it helps mental health, as well as physical health, of course. Have you thought about other ways of moving more without a gym membership? Exercising outdoors may be even more effective because morning daylight can help our mood and sleep.

We can help to identify specific small steps,

What would be a first small way you could include some movement in your day? Walking to the park and eating lunch there sounds like a great idea.

We can **educate** about sleep and **encourage** healthier habits,

Good sleep is important for mood. Using tablets or phones or screens of any sort at bedtime can interfere with the quality of sleep because the blue light from the screens tells the brain, "See the light and the blue sky. It's morning! Time to be awake and get up!" which is not helpful when you are trying to sleep. Reading and responding to social media or the news stimulates the brain even more and puts it in work mode rather than rest mode.

Would you consider changing this use of your phone? What would your plan be? When would you stop using your phone? Where would you leave it to charge?

Elephants are things that might feel big or awkward to discuss – we may try to ignore them or skirt around them. The risk of this is that we don't leave enough time to address them properly. We may delay or avoid this topic, even if it could be a crucial part of improving someone's health. If we notice situations when we are reluctant to bring up an issue, then we might practice with a colleague to gain confidence, for example,

This can be difficult to talk about because we might not be used to discussing it but, in health, we we always ask people about… alcohol / drug use / thoughts of self-harm or suicide.

Additional tasks for the health professional within clinical management

There are other things we may do apart from the 5Es. We might try some of the following.

Reflect a strength

During data gathering, we may have heard particular strengths, and there may be unseen or unharnessed strengths as well. Sometimes, we may need to reframe these – to describe them in a slightly different way that shifts perspective,

It took courage to come and see me today – well done.

It takes strength to open up and show your feelings through crying. I'm so pleased you felt able to do so.

You succeeded at getting an appointment with me – and that's not always easy, is it? Your persistence and tenacity paid off.

Use a metaphor

These can help explain and illustrate what we think is going on and why. One metaphor is the oars of a boat. What do we mean by oars? We use oars to row a boat, to move it from one place to another. We use oars as a metaphor for the tools or resources that a person can use to move themselves from a place where they are stuck, towards a goal. See Chapter 5.

During data gathering, we have listened to and learnt the patient's own "oars" – the tools they are currently using. These will be different for everyone. In clinical management, we can ask, *What do you think could be another oar to add in?* Remember to pause and listen rather than provide the answer.

Small steps

The health professional can help with being realistic about small, manageable steps that someone can start.

Getting from where someone is now to where they want or need to be may feel so daunting that it seems impossible. A journey from Lands End to John o'Groats – the whole length of Britain – might feel absolutely impossible. It's 600 miles. But, every year, people do it, and many people who wouldn't even contemplate a long-distance walk do cover 5 miles in a day – which is 35 miles a week. Four months of daily 5-mile walks would complete a 600-mile journey.

In the same way, we need to help people start the journey towards better mental health by thinking about small positive steps – something they could do today or tomorrow and keep doing.

If someone is stuck with inertia and does not know which direction to take, we can think of a small step in **any** direction. It does not have to be the right direction; the important thing is to stop being stuck and get started. If the first step turns out to be in the wrong direction, we still have movement and momentum, so it is easier to keep going and change direction.

How do we make sure that someone is committed to an action? We could ask specific leading questions:

Does that feel like something you could do?

Does it feel manageable?

Can we agree that as a plan?

What day will you start to do this?

Grow the team

Discuss how to "grow the team" – identifying and harnessing the support of useful people around the person – friends, relatives, work colleagues and other professionals.

Where we sense that people have little support, we may want to help them to grow their team. During data gathering, we have found out who is in their life and we have listened for people offering support, whether they are friends, partners or work colleagues. It may be helpful to identify a "go-to" person:

Who could you phone if you feel really bad – your mum or your sister?

Who else could help – who is on your side? How can we involve them?

How could you contact this person/these people?

Throughout clinical management, we listen as well as talk and reflect back what we hear, encouraging and nudging where we can, working in partnership with the person. The plan should be an agreed and shared strategy, not something that is "delivered" to them. Genuinely shared management is far more likely to be put into action.

Coping questions

If we have asked coping questions and found out what the person is doing now that is helping them to cope, then we can encourage them to continue with this and perhaps develop it further, e.g. discuss increasing the number of times an activity takes place in a week.

Paperwork and prescriptions

We can discuss whether being at work is helpful and indeed therapeutic, providing a sense of purpose, a structure to the daily routine and an opportunity to be with others. Or perhaps work is increasing stress and it may be appropriate to take time off or request amended hours or duties at work.

We may decide if any investigations are indicated or referrals are needed.

Medication

There are times when it will be appropriate to prescribe medication using evidence-based guidance, such as from the UK National Institute for Clinical Excellence (NICE) or Clinical Knowledge Summaries (CKS), or local pathways.

Resources

We may provide written material such as patient information about mental health problems from patient.info or cci.health.wa.gov.au.

There is an almost overwhelming number of online resources and apps for mental health. There are ones that are suited to particular conditions, aimed at specific ages, designed more as games or more fact-based. Some can be personalised and may link with primary care notes. Online CBT may be a way to access timely help but might be limited by factors such as motivation, internet connection and an appropriate device.

Confirm a shared management plan and next steps

How do we know when we have an agreed plan? We are looking for a "yes" – a set of responses that tells us that the person is in agreement and minded to do what we have talked about and shared with them. At this point, if we are on the right track, everything about the patient will be saying "yes" – words, tone of voice and non-verbal cues are all congruently positive.

Safety netting

It is always worth discussing what to do if things are getting worse, whether by briefly mentioning this and providing a 24/7 phone support number or a more in-depth plan.

A safety net should involve a plan appropriate to the consultation – one that flows naturally from the conversation and is empowering, not terrifying. Straightforward consultations may not need a safety net, so think whether this is necessary. If one is needed, think of it as a three-part structure:[2]

> *This is what I, [the health professional], expect to happen* – This is where we, as clinicians, share an appropriate amount of knowledge about the natural history and evolution of problems, using language that is patient-friendly, i.e. not jargon words or acronyms. This is a time to be lay-person friendly, inform and educate, not to be a "clever health professional"; we share our thought process.

> *This is how you will know if I'm wrong* – It is empowering for a person to know that whilst we hope we are right, we acknowledge that we may have got it wrong or something unexpected might happen.

> *This is what you should do then* – This is again educational and also reassuring – empowering the person so that they know what to do if the unexpected happens.

Follow up

What is going to happen next? How can the primary care team check in on progress? When starting out in primary care or using a new approach, proactively following up is a great way to understand what has been helpful and what you might change in the future.

The final part of management is to think when and under what circumstances we want to see the person again. This might be "if" or "when" – conditional or unconditional. It may be that we want to see someone if particular circumstances happen:

> *If you are not feeling much better in a couple of weeks.*

> *If you are still feeling anxious despite doing what we have discussed.*

If things start to get worse.

Or, particularly in mental health consultations, we might want to see someone regardless, offering an unconditional follow-up,

I'd like to see you in two weeks to see how you are getting on, putting into practice what we have discussed today. If you speak to reception, they will be able to book you in.

Wherever possible, be specific – clear about the circumstances that should make someone return and clear about how to book that appointment or telephone call with you.

Why shouldn't I just prescribe? After all, if the patient is depressed, they need antidepressants, don't they?

A review of the literature,[3] found that the evidence for using antidepressants for patients with mild–moderate depression was weak and concluded that psychological therapies should be used first. Antidepressants may be used later, but only if active monitoring and other treatments have failed.

Responding to unrealistic requests

Here are some commonly heard phrases and the ways we may respond to them,

- *I need something to make me happy.*

    Sometimes, for some people, medication may have a role alongside other things to help change mood, but there is no "happy pill".

- *I want to forget about what happened.*

    It was a very upsetting event but, unfortunately, there is no "delete" for any thought, feeling or memory, but there are ways this can change or feel easier.

- *I just want to turn my brain off.*

    Even though it can appeal when we feel overwhelmed and exhausted, the brain keeps going, but there are ways to train your brain to feel calmer.

Key points – be a safe clinician and consider physical and mental health overlaps

Many people experiencing physical symptoms will understandably also be anxious, stressed or have low mood. There are shared physiological, lifestyle and environmental factors that create overlaps between some physical and mental health conditions, particularly diabetes or heart disease and depression. Some factors that may contribute to these physical and mental health pathologies include disrupted sleep, inflammation, a sedentary lifestyle and diet.

Always ask yourself what physical health problems need to be investigated, managed or excluded rather than managing a mental health problem in isolation. Use tools to manage stress and anxiety alongside investigation or referral, but consider each person holistically and take care not to make assumptions that mean physical illness is missed.

Keep in mind:

- Women in their late 30s and older who feel irritable and anxious, with sleep issues or reduced libido, may be experiencing the perimenopause rather than a primary mental health diagnosis.
- Chronic fatigue syndrome may have symptoms that overlap with depression and other mental health issues, but the management will be different.
- Metabolic disorders are common in those on antipsychotics, and regular assessment for cardiovascular disease is a priority in those with chronic mental health diagnoses.
- Physical and mental health conditions with similar symptoms can co-exist – for example, someone with a long-standing bipolar diagnosis may present with new onset of hyperthyroidism.

References

1. Blount, E., Kirby-Blount, H., & Moulton, L. (2021). The Complete MRCGP Casebook: 100 Consultations for the RCA/CSA across the NEW 2020 RCGP Curriculum (2nd ed.). CRC Press. https://doi.org/10.1201/9781003110729
2. Neighbour, R. (2005). The Inner Consultation: How to Develop an Effective and Intuitive Consulting Style (2nd ed.). CRC Press. https://doi.org/10.1201/9780203736548
3. Arroll, B., Moir, F., & Kendrick, T. (2017). Effective Management of Depression in Primary Care: A Review of the Literature. BJGP Open. https://doi.org/10.3399%2Fbjgpopen17X101025

Mental health and the GP curriculum

It would be difficult to find a country with a primary care curriculum that does not include mental health and, of course, it is one of the 20 clinical curriculum areas of the RCGP. It is a particularly important and significant area, as mental health problems are very common in primary care and include people from all age groups.

Mental health impacts right across the curriculum domains. Considering the RCGP clinical experience groups, it is easy to see how almost all of them may include mental health issues.

Infants, children and young people – child and adolescent mental health problems, including neurological and developmental disorders.

Gender, reproductive and sexual health – the antenatal, intranatal and postnatal periods are times of increased risk. Those who identify as LGBTQIA+ also have a higher risk of developing mental health problems.

People with long-term conditions – long-term conditions and chronic pain overlap considerably with mental health problems. People with serious or significant mental health problems are more at risk of developing long-term conditions such as diabetes and cardiovascular disease.

Older adults – may develop any mental health problems. Anxiety and depression may be early symptoms of dementia. Some illnesses that predominantly affect older adults, such as Parkinson's disease, frequently include depression as a key symptom.

DOI: 10.1201/9781003409168-5

Urgent and unscheduled care – management of acute mental health problems such as psychosis, suicide risk and presentations with big emotions.

People with health disadvantages and vulnerabilities – including veterans, refugees and migrants who may experience mental health problems such as PTSD. Many health and socioeconomic disadvantages may put people at greater risk of developing mental health problems.

Population health and health promotion – encouraging mental well-being and resilience.

And, of course,

Mental health, including addiction, alcohol and substance misuse.

What is mental health and how does it fit with primary care?

Mental health is defined[1] as a state of well-being in which individuals can:

- Realise their potential.
- Cope with the normal stress of everyday life.
- Work productively and fruitfully.
- Contribute to their community.

Primary mental health care means:

- First-line interventions that are provided as an integral part of general health care.
- Mental health care provided by primary care workers who are skilled, able and supported to provide mental health services.

There are strong arguments as to why mental health care should be integrated into primary care. Mental health problems are very common: 1 in 6 adults and 1 in 10 children are likely to have a mental health problem in any 12-month period. It is estimated that 30% of people who see their GP have a mental health component to their illness.[2]

Primary care services are efficient and generally directly accessible to patients. Primary care for mental health problems is effective and highly cost-effective. In the UK, more than 90% of these patients are cared for entirely within primary care – and yet primary care uses less than 10% of the total mental health expenditure.

The RCGP reminds us that an average UK GP list of 2,000 patients will have people experiencing the following:[2]

- Common mental health problems – 352 people.
- Sub-threshold common mental health problems – a further 352 people.
- Personality disorder – 176 people.
- Long-term physical health condition with additional mental health problem – 125 people.
- Alcohol dependency – 120 people.
- Sub-threshold psychosis – 120 people.
- Medically unexplained symptoms – 100 people.
- Drug dependency – 60 people.
- Psychosis – 8 people.

How do people with mental health problems or distress present in primary care?

Sometimes people present to us with symptoms that immediately suggest a mental health problem, for example:

- Feeling low in mood, depressed, anxious or angry.
- Poor concentration.
- Self-harming.
- Thought disorders.
- Tearfulness.
- Psychomotor agitation or retardation.
- Sleep disturbance – can't get to sleep, early morning waking, night terrors.

However, other people present symptoms that they experience elsewhere in their bodies, for example the following:

Gastrointestinal

- Loss of appetite, bloating, discomfort, altered bowel habit, constipation and diarrhoea.

Cardiovascular

- Chest tightness, palpitations and awareness of heartbeat.

Sexual health

- Changes to the menstrual cycle, including secondary amenorrhoea.
- Loss of libido.

General

- Feeling tired all the time.
- Unexplained aches and pains.

Psychosocial

- Avoiding contact with friends and family.
- Neglecting hobbies or other interests.
- Experiencing problems at home, work or in family life.

Of course, we must consider the possibility of significant physical illness and investigate appropriately. But, having done so, unless there are new symptoms or signs, then repeated investigation may be unhelpful. It may reinforce the idea that there is something physical to be found and may not be the best use of resources. A transdiagnostic approach may then be preferable – assessing the person in front of us and the problems they present, without separating "physical" problems to investigate and manage from "mental" health problems.

What is the role of the primary care clinician?

The RCGP describes the following:[3]

- **Clinical management** – including diagnosis, investigation and referral if appropriate.
- **Communication** – with patients, relatives and carers.
- **Risk assessment** – clinician, patient, others. This includes early intervention such as referral where appropriate, safety netting, follow-up and continuity of care.
- **Coordination of care** – including with the Community Mental Health Trust (CMHT), social workers, the ambulance service, secondary care, the voluntary sector and the police. Use protocols such as the Mental Health Act (MHA) and Mental Capacity Act (MCA) where appropriate.

- **Empower patients and carers** – prevention, prescribing, monitoring and self-management of both mental and physical multimorbidity.
- **Remember physical health problems** – patients with a primary diagnosis of a mental health problem are just as likely as everyone else to develop physical illness and more likely to be at risk of cardiovascular disease and diabetes.

The areas of data gathering and clinical management have been considered in depth in Chapters 1 and 2. As an overview, the following are some of the tasks to complete within a mental health consultation.

Data gathering and making a diagnosis

- How is the patient presenting the problem? Is this a typical or atypical presentation?
- What are their thoughts and their worries about this problem?
- Who is this person in the context of their life – home, relationships, work, hobbies, etc.?
- What are their risk factors – lifestyle, cultural, socioeconomic, family history, etc.?
- What are the red flags?
- What relevant investigations are needed?
- How do we interpret test results?
- What is the differential diagnosis?

Clinical management and complexity

Aspects of management

What can we do in primary care?

- Initial management today – which might sometimes include emergency management.
- Continuing care.
- Chronic disease support.
- Patient education – directly and via information leaflets or web links.

What can the person do for themselves?

- Self-help measures.
- Self-referral to counselling.

What can other people help us with? Do we need to involve:

- Others in the primary healthcare team.
- Mental health services.

Patient care pathways

Do we know how the following pathways work in our area?

- How do primary, secondary and community care join up?
- How are these pathways accessed by professionals and patients?
- What self-referral pathways are available for self-help, support groups or counselling?
- How are transitions of care managed? For example, how does a young person move from child to adult mental health services?

The RCGP assessment tools

Given the importance of mental health in the GP curriculum, it is unsurprising that this area is assessed in various ways and using different assessment tools.

Workplace-based assessment

The mental health curriculum can be assessed through most of the tools for workplace-based assessment, for example:

- CAT – the care assessment tool is used to discuss patients presenting with mental health problems. This might be through random case analysis, case-based discussion, referrals review or other variants.
- COT and audio COT – the consultation observation tool can be used to assess performance in this area of the curriculum.
- QIA/QIP – we may think of undertaking a quality improvement activity or project to audit or improve the care of people with mental health problems.

Link appropriate learning logs and assessments to the clinical experience group "Mental health (including addiction, alcohol and drug abuse)". This will form part of the whole picture of curriculum coverage, ready for assessment at Annual Review of Competency Progression (ARCP) in due course.

Applied Knowledge Test (AKT)

The AKT is a multiple-choice exam of 200 questions to be answered in 3 hours and 10 minutes. Of these questions, 80% relate to clinical knowledge, 10% are evidence-based practice and 10% concern primary care management. Within the 160 clinical knowledge questions, expect a significant proportion to include mental health issues. The RCGP curriculum gives the following examples of what might be tested in the AKT:

- Symptoms of schizophrenia.
- Increased health risk of atypical antipsychotic drugs.
- CBT in anxiety management.

Consultation skills assessment

In the consultation skills assessment exam, there is likely to be at least one patient with a problem that is primarily related to mental health and others where there are mental health symptoms or problems that are adding complexity. Again, some examples from the RCGP curriculum include the following:

- A woman has ongoing abdominal pain, and the gastroenterology letter (provided) indicates no organic cause.
- A young mother is worried by thoughts that TV and radio presenters are talking about her, despite acknowledging that this cannot logically be the case.
- A teenager asks for help with compulsive tidying, which takes hours and interferes with his schoolwork.

Summary and conclusion

Mental health problems are very common and may present to primary care in a variety of different ways.

The RCGP curriculum appropriately covers a wide range of mental health problems and presentations. This is an important learning area for GPs and other primary care health professionals.

In this book, we share tools to use in a variety of mental health and addiction problems. Using these can help your development as a skilled practitioner in primary mental healthcare, able to empower patients.

References

1. World Health Organization and World Organization of Family Doctors (Wonca). (2008). Integrating Mental Health into Primary Care: A Global Perspective.
2. RCGP Position Statement on Mental Health in Primary Care. (2017). https://www.rcgp.org.uk/representing-you/policy-areas/mental-health-in-primary-care [accessed 17 May 2023].
3. RCGP Curriculum for Mental Health. (2017). https://www.rcgp.org.uk/mrcgp-exams/gp-curriculum/clinical-topic-guides#mental [accessed 17 May 2023].

4

The theory behind the practice

Mental health models – introduction

In this chapter, we describe and explain some of the theories and models that underpin the practical tools in this book. We are busy primary care practitioners, and we want to be able to make a difference to patients within a time-limited primary care consultation. Longer therapies are for others, for example clinical psychologists and counsellors, who typically provide 50 minutes for each patient. However, we can borrow from these in-depth tools in our own brief consultations.

For those who would like to learn more, there are references and further reading at the end of the chapter. Courses covering cognitive behavioural therapy (CBT), acceptance commitment therapy (ACT), motivational interviewing (MI) and others are available, and additional skills in these areas may be very useful in day-to-day clinical work.

Each model described in this chapter may be used as a "very brief psychological intervention". What does this mean? There are some components of accepted, evidence-based, longer-term interventions and:

- They are very brief, for example only one encounter or delivered within a short time frame rather than regular sessions over weeks or months.
- They can be, and are, delivered by people with less specialised training, for example primary healthcare professionals rather than psychotherapists or psychiatrists.

DOI: 10.1201/9781003409168-6

Many primary care health professionals will experience a time when they have said to a patient something as brief as, *With your goal of improving your health, stopping smoking would be the best thing you could do*, and the patient has done exactly that – an effective intervention that took a mere three seconds.

In this chapter, we will briefly describe a number of the core psychological models used currently and influencing this text:

- CBT.
- Behavioural activation.
- Graded exposure.
- MI.
- ACT.
- Focused ACT (FACT).
- Positive psychology.
- Using metaphor.
- Transactional analysis.

Cognitive behavioural therapy

CBT, developed by Aaron Beck,[1] is based on the idea that it is not so much the situation itself that disturbs us but our interpretation of it. This interpretation influences our thoughts, emotions and behaviours, creating a vicious negative cycle.

It is one of the most studied forms of psychotherapy and is used extensively. There is evidence for its effectiveness in many conditions, and it can be used in different modalities, such as e-CBT.

The second wave of CBT added an understanding of broader aspects affecting mental health, including factors such as race and poverty. A five-part model was introduced as a simple tool to help patients understand how CBT works. The five parts are situation, thinking, emotions, behaviour and physical sensations.[2]

CBT is based on three levels of thinking:

1 **Automatic thoughts** – in depression: *I am a burden to others; I will never get better.*

2 **Rules for living** (underlying assumptions): *Only weak people get depressed* and, commonly, *If I tell people what I am feeling, then I will be rejected.*

3 **Core beliefs** – may be helpful or unhelpful:

Helpful: *I am lovable.*
Unhelpful: *I am weak.*

In depression, unhelpful core beliefs may predominate. In anxiety disorders, the dominant core belief may be *I am out of control.*

Here is an example of the five-part model of CBT, depicted in Figure 4.1:[3,4]

1 **Situation or environment** – where we are and what is happening.
2 **Thoughts** – our internal running commentary.
3 **Feelings** – emotional responses such as fear and guilt.
4 **Action/behaviours** – the things we do or don't do.
5 **Physiology** – bodily changes such as heart racing, sweaty palms, shaking.

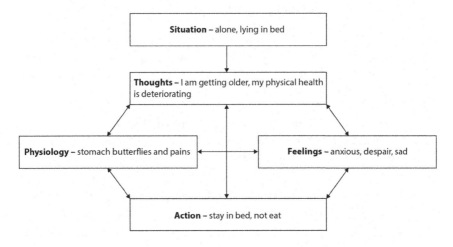

FIGURE 4.1 Five-part CBT model example.[2]

For example, if I am,

1 Lying alone in bed.
2 I might start thinking about my physical health problems and dwelling on how I am getting old.

3 I might then feel sad and low, afraid for my future, anxious and in despair.

4 This might mean I don't bother getting up, or I eat poor food and don't exercise.

5 I might then notice stomach butterflies and pains and think about my physical health and how my body is getting old and frail.

How does CBT work?

Working within a 5-part model, CBT aims to stop these vicious cycles by changing one of the components. This could be replacing the **thought**. Alternatively, planning a **behavioural change**, such as a daily walk to the end of the street, or a change aimed at **physiological responses**, such as, *When I notice this happening, I will spend one minute focusing on breathing.* It is virtually impossible to make a plan to **feel** differently. This is worth remembering, as it can explain why it is difficult to know what to suggest, when someone tells us, *I just want to feel happy and relaxed.* We need to shift this conversation to consider the thoughts, behaviours and physiological changes that will accompany and promote this feeling.

At each consultation, we may check in with the patient, using the five-part model, to see how the vicious cycle may be reversing. This provides motivation for patients and the "empirical evidence" that Beck introduced to CBT – that the person is their own "scientist".

One aim of CBT is that it becomes **self-sustainable**. This means that lessons learnt can be applied to other situations in the future, developing the person's resilience and adaptive responses to their everyday world.

Using questions in CBT to encourage reflection and problem-solving

In CBT, we may use a Socratic style of questioning to encourage reflection and problem-solving. This also helps build rapport and maintains the active involvement and motivation of the patient in their recovery. We can support someone to think through their current problems and find solutions that have helped in the past or when they have felt less distress. The four stages are:

1 Asking open questions to understand their world, *What do you mean when you say you "feel depressed"?*

2 Empathic and attentive listening.

3   Frequent summarising.

4   Asking the person to synthesise and analyse the new information about their current problem, *Is there a different point of view?*

We may reflect back, repeating key words used in the same tone (simple reflection) or rephrasing to capture meaning (complex reflection). Regular reflections with a concluding summary provide opportunities to check in and to ensure there is mutual understanding and a plan for the next activity (the homework of CBT).

In this approach, we do not tell the person what to do but use this style of questioning to help them think through their problems. If they are stuck, we may suggest how others have overcome their distress.

Behavioural activation

Behavioural activation, which is part of CBT, recognises that there are things we do that affect how we feel. In depression, we may stop or avoid doing things, but if we go ahead regardless, we may find our mood improves as a consequence.

Behavioural activation originates from behavioural psychology. This states that the way we behave is due to our environment and is a conditioned response. Activities that fulfil us or lead to happiness are more likely to be repeated. Conversely, if activities result in unpleasant feelings, we are less likely to do them or anything else. The worse we feel, the less we do – a vicious spiral downwards. How can we apply this principle?

- **Increasing pleasure**. Perhaps we enjoy walking and feel good after a long walk. If we are experiencing low mood or depression, we may not feel motivated to go walking. If, however, we plan to go for a very short walk each day regardless of motivation, then we may notice our mood improve.

- **Replacing unhelpful behaviours**. Perhaps we use alcohol to wind down when tense and stressed but then sleep poorly, wake up tired and are less able to cope with the stress. In this situation, we might consciously choose to replace using alcohol with something else to de-stress, for example physical exercise such as a boxing class at the gym.

- **Improving relationships**. When we feel down, we may not bother as much with helpful relationships with friends or family. We may spend more time alone with thoughts that make loneliness or depression worse. How can we break this cycle? It can help to commit to manageable regular social contacts that are small and achievable and notice how we think and feel afterwards.

Graded exposure

Exposure therapy is an intervention that emerged from CBT. It is a psychological tool that is particularly useful when someone has a specific anxiety that results in the avoidance of people, places or objects. It offers a way to gradually build up to a desired activity, moving through negotiated manageable actions. It could be considered like a step ladder where the top rung is the situation or activity causing the anxiety. Lower rungs cause less anxiety. Step by step, and over time, the person can gradually extinguish the high levels of anxiety by facing their fear.

Motivational interviewing[5,6]

MI was developed to help people break away from life-changing negative habits such as alcohol addiction. Like CBT, it adopts a collaborative, person-centred approach that aims to create and maintain motivation, enhancing autonomy and improving someone's capacity to make changes in their life.

MI nudges towards change. It does more than simply listening well, but less than directing or telling someone what they should do. It adopts a position of equals, with people feeling respected and empowered to make changes they may have felt incapable of doing. MI is particularly useful when there are one or more of the following:

- **Ambivalence** – *I have mixed feelings about change. On the one hand… but on the other hand….*
- **Lack of confidence** – *I'm not actually sure if I can change….*
- **Lack of desire** – *I don't know if I want to.*
- **Low priority/importance** – the advantages of change and the disadvantages of the status quo are unclear.

To make changes, we must be "ready, willing and able":

- **Ready** – it's a priority.
- **Willing** – it's important to change.
- **Able** – have the confidence to change.

Techniques in MI follow the style of Socratic questioning described earlier and will be familiar to anyone who has learnt consultation skills. They include:

- Attentive listening using open questions to understand what is important.
- Building rapport.
- Affirming and reinforcing positive behaviour.
- Reflections – both simple and more complex, where we rephrase to capture the meaning.
- Summary – to check there is mutual understanding.

It is often an iterative process. A "failure" is harnessed as an opportunity to revisit the above tools and to reflect together on how to make and sustain lasting change.

Acceptance and commitment therapy[7,8]

Third-wave CBT therapies, such as dialectical behavioural therapy (DBT) and ACT, expand on traditional CBT. They use a holistic approach to develop mental flexibility for times when we feel stuck. Rather than the contents of our thoughts, the focus is on how a person relates to the thought.

DBT focuses on interpersonal relationships and the emotional and social aspects of living. It is composed of four modules: mindfulness, distress tolerance, emotional regulation and interpersonal effectiveness.

ACT starts with the premise that psychological discomfort and pain are an integral part of life and uses mindfulness to help us stay in the present moment, accepting thoughts and feelings without judging them. It differs from CBT in that it does not seek to change unpleasant thoughts or feelings but rather seeks to help patients learn to co-exist with them. There are six core principles:

1 **Acceptance** – an active choice to allow unpleasant thoughts or feelings to co-exist rather than trying to distract ourselves from them or fight or try to forget them.

2 **Cognitive defusion** – rather than being caught up inside a thought, we separate ourselves and look at the thoughts. Rather than believing that we are totally helpless, we could notice that our brain has become caught up in the thought of being helpless.

3 **Being present** – as in mindfulness, being present in the here-and-now, for example being consciously aware of our bodies through breathing exercises.

4 **Self as context** – we are more than our current feelings and thoughts. There is a "self" outside this. However much I worry, it does not define me as "a worried person"; instead, it is reframed as, *I experience feelings of worry.*

5 **Values** – what really matters to us? When we understand the things that are most important to us, we can use these to provide direction for our actions.

6 **Committed action** – can we use our values as a compass to take meaningful action, even while there may be thoughts or feelings that make this task feel difficult? ACT suggests that we do something every day that is congruent with our values.

Many people will have heard of the "acceptance prayer" attributed to Niebuhr (1943), which has many versions, but neatly expresses the principles of ACT,

> *Give me grace to accept with serenity the things that cannot be changed, courage to change the things which should be changed, and the wisdom to distinguish the one from the other. Living one day at a time, enjoying one moment at a time, accepting hardship as a pathway to peace.*

Focused acceptance and commitment therapy (FACT)

In general, ACT is seen as a therapy used by psychologists and therapists over several or many 50-minute therapy sessions. FACT refers to a briefer form that can readily be used in a primary care consultation. The reference[9] at the end of this chapter links to a video demonstrating its use in a brief consultation.

Positive psychology

In medicine, we often start with problems and then look for solutions. In positive psychology, we start with strengths. Instead of looking for emotional weaknesses, we look for assets and resources that someone is already using and build on and develop these to enhance mental well-being. A simple example of this might be a gratitude list.

In this situation, we are not looking for problems, worries, challenges or difficulties but are looking at the positives. For example,

What are you thankful for in your life?

Who are you grateful to?

What was the best thing that happened today?

What was the nicest thing you ate today?

What did you see or do outside today?

The act of thinking about and writing down these positive thoughts encourages reflection and reinforces them. In turn, we might show gratitude to others and, through reflecting and practising gratitude and positivity, we may develop our skills to increase that positivity.

Using metaphor

In the third wave of CBT, Padesky and Mooney introduced resilience and resourcefulness as a new component of CBT.[10] To prepare someone for discharge from formal therapy, they used metaphor and analogy to provide examples to encourage endurance and "stickability" of new skills. CBT provides a way to see ourselves, others or a situation differently; for example, looking at a five-part model may bring a richer understanding of why a person felt compelled to leave a stressful situation, and what could be worked on to change this in the future.

Metaphors align with mental health because they function as a connection and provide a comparison between a subject that feels hard to understand and one that is familiar. Metaphors help us to organise our experiences and learn, hence their use in medicine, where we describe unseen physiological concepts in familiar terms such as, *the heart is a pump pushing blood around the pipes of the body.*

There is research into the use of metaphors in health care. Looking at doctors' communication skills, Casarett et al.[11] explored how 94 patients with advanced cancer rated the effectiveness of their doctors' abilities to talk to them. They analysed a total of 101 consultations and coded these for metaphor and analogy content. Overall, those doctors who used more metaphors elicited higher patient ratings for effective communication. Within the field of mental health, there has been interest in the use of metaphor and its potential as a part of a therapeutic intervention, described in the book on CBT and metaphor.[12]

In psychological practice, metaphors may form part of the core intervention. Sims (2003)[13] developed a six-stage model in which a metaphor that is used by a patient is identified, validated and worked with by expanding the metaphor and connecting it with the future.

Transactional analysis

Transactional analysis is a psychoanalytical theory whereby social interactions (transactions) are examined, and the "ego state" is used as a way to understand the interaction. Eric Berne[14] described how the human psyche has three different states. These three states are parent, adult and child. Each of us has all three states, and we move between them according to the situation we find ourselves in, though we may notice tendencies towards certain states in certain interactions:

- **Parent** – can be caring and nurturing but can also be punitive and controlling. The parent may "judge" and use words like "should" or "should not".
- **Adult** – makes everyday decisions almost without thinking, for example always having a cup of tea for the first drink of the day, so freeing up brain space for executive functioning and significant decisions.
- **Child** – may be spontaneous and creative but could also be whining and manipulative or helpless.

In general, adult–adult communication will be most effective. During a conversation, the following can indicate that at least one person, or both, has left the adult state:

- It is not going as we intended.
- We feel uncomfortable.
- We are struggling to communicate.

After the conversation, we may reflect and wonder why **we** responded as we did.

OK/Not OK matrix

The OK/not OK principle (Figure 4.2) comes from transactional analysis. There are four basic life positions from which we can see ourselves and others.

The "I am OK, you are OK" position is considered optimal and, in this position, we hold the belief that all people are valuable and accepted. This belief will mean we believe that people can solve their problems and we can partner together as equals. Being non-judgemental and curious, even with someone who is encountering objective difficulties, indicates our belief that "I am OK, you are OK".

If we believe "I am OK, you are not OK", we may find that without consciously intending it, we act in ways that are judgemental or create a hierarchy between the people in the conversation, where we imply "I am better than you" because of my state of being "OK". If we encounter someone who seems continually angry or critical, it could be that they have this position. The "I am not OK, you are OK" similarly creates a power hierarchy, but in this case, the person with this position may continually put others' needs before their own and see themselves as the victim.

I'm not OK You're OK	I'm OK You're OK
I'm not OK You're not OK	I'm OK You're not OK

FIGURE 4.2 OK/not OK matrix.

Key points – theory

There are a number of theoretical models that are extensively researched and widely used in treating mental health conditions such as worry, stress and anxiety. While these can seem daunting to undertake, there are aspects of these theories that can be translated to a primary care context and be applicable to daily mental health conversations.

Almost all of these theories and therapies can be traced back to or linked with CBT, making it the biggest influence on this text.

References

CBT

1. Beck, A.T. (1976). Cognitive Therapy and the Emotional Disorders. International Universities Press.
2. International Cognitive Therapy Newsletter. (1990). Clinical Tip Presenting the Cognitive Model to Client. Volume 6 – includes Volumes 5(2) and 6(1&2). Editor: Kathleen A. Mooney, Ph.D.; Associate Editor: Christine A. Padesky, Ph.D.
3. Williams, C.J. (2001). Overcoming Depression: A Five Areas Approach. Arnold.
4. Williams, C., & Garland, A. (2002). A Cognitive-Behavioural Therapy Assessment Model for Use in Everyday Clinical Practice. Adv Psychiatr Treat. 8(2): 172–9.

Motivational interviewing

5. https://motivationalinterviewing.org/understanding-motivational-interviewing
6. https://www.racgp.org.au/afp/2012/september/motivational-interviewing-techniques [accessed 19 May 2023].

ACT and FACT

7. https://positivepsychology.com/act-acceptance-and-commitment-therapy/ [accessed 13 November 2022].
8. https://www.sbsaba.com/applying-the-six-core-act-processes-during-the-current-pandemic-crisis/ [accessed 13 November 2022].
9. https://www.healthnavigator.org.nz/clinicians/f/fact-therapy/ [accessed 13 November 2022]. It includes a link to a video demonstrating the use of FACT in an 11-minute consultation.

Metaphor

10. Padesky CA, Mooney KA. (2012) Strengths-based cognitive-behavioural therapy: a four-step model to build resilience. Clin Psychol Psychother. Jul-Aug;19(4):283–90.
11. Casarett, D., Pickard, A., Fishman, J.M., Alexander, S.C., Arnold, R.M., Pollak, K.I., & Tulsky, J.A. (2010). Can metaphors and analogies improve communication with seriously ill patients? J Palliat Med. 13(3):255–60. https://doi.org/10.1089/jpm.2009.0221
12. Stott, R., Mansell, W., Salkovskis, P., Lavender, A., & Cartwright-Hatton, S. (2010). Oxford Guide to Metaphors in CBT: Building Cognitive Bridges. Oxford University Press.
13. Sims, P.A.(2003). Working with metaphor. Am J Psychother. 57(4):528–36. doi: 10.1176/appi.psychotherapy.2003.57.4.528.

Transactional analysis

14. Berne, E. (1964). Games People Play – The Basic Hand Book of Transactional Analysis. Ballantine Books.

Further reading

General

Roberts, K., Travers-Hill, E., Coker, S., Troup, J., Casey, S., Parkin, K., et al. (2021). Brief Psychological Interventions for Anxiety and Depression in a Secondary Care Adult Mental Health Service: An Evaluation. Cogn Behav Ther. 14:e29.

Behavioural activation

https://www.medicalnewstoday.com/articles/behavioral-activation#examples [accessed 26 May 2023].

CBT

https://cogbtherapy.com/cbt-model-of-emotions [accessed 26 May 2023].

5

Sharing understanding using metaphors

Introduction – what is a metaphor?

A metaphor is a way of describing something in a way that isn't literally true but helps us make better sense of the issue. We may use metaphors to help depict or explain something that is otherwise complex or hard to describe. Metaphor literally means "to transfer" – so we may perhaps transfer a thought, description or feeling from one world to another.

A recent example is "Waging war on COVID-19". We could, of course, describe the challenges, logistics and complexities of virus sequencing, vaccine production, roll-out programmes, disease surveillance and the worry of virus mutation – but using the phrase "waging war" gives us an image that is easy to understand. Even if we have not lived through a war, we have seen war on television or in films and can transfer the concept of fighting a hostile enemy that is attacking us and our society to the complexities of managing a new and deadly illness.

When do we use metaphors and why?

We often use metaphors in everyday life, possibly without realising,

She's on an emotional roller coaster.

I'm an early bird but you're a night owl.

The twins are two peas in a pod.

DOI: 10.1201/9781003409168-7

You should turn a blind eye.

I've got cold feet about that interview.

And, of course, our patients sometimes communicate their feelings and experiences through metaphor.

METAPHOR	POSSIBLE MEANING
I saw red	I was very angry
I blew my top	I was shouting at everyone
I've got the blues	I'm feeling sad/low/depressed
I'm down in the dumps	I'm feeling sad/low/depressed
I need to let off steam	I'm under a lot of pressure
Everything is weighing me down	I'm overburdened/low/not coping
I'm wading through treacle	Everything is an effort, really hard
I'm a bag of nerves	I feel anxious
I'm beginning to rattle	I seem to be taking a lot of tablets

We can use metaphors in at least three different ways to help our communication:

- **Naming** – when we need to describe body parts, symptoms or functions in a way that is comprehensible.
- **Framing** – to help someone perceive the problem differently.
- **Motivation** – to help persuade someone to change their behaviour.

The use of metaphor may in itself be therapeutic. It enables us to use imagination and creativity to understand ourselves and the world, improve self-regard and encourage positive change.

Why do we use metaphors in mental health conversations?

Metaphors can help with learning and understanding, and an image can be easy to remember. Using metaphor can also enhance rapport and strengthen the therapeutic relationship. It may also introduce a small but helpful element of fun or humour to lighten a conversation.

Particularly if we share similar backgrounds and a common language, metaphor can be a concise and easy way to demonstrate to someone that we understand what they are saying.

Example – someone tells us how difficult life is for them and how hard it is to get anything done.

We might say – *You're wading through treacle.*

It can help make an invisible problem more visible and understandable.

Example – someone is telling us about how apprehensive they are about a vague and rather nebulous future filled with dread.

We might say – *The skies are grey and storm clouds are gathering.*

Or we can use metaphors to de-medicalise and avoid jargon in explanations.

Example – we want to explain why it is difficult for someone with depression to get motivated and do anything.

We might say – *Lots of things are weighing you down. If we can start to lift some of these weights from you, it will become easier for you to start doing things that are important to you. Let's think how we could do that – even removing a small weight will help.*

Who might particularly benefit from the use of metaphor?

Some people are what we call "psychologically minded" – they understand mood and emotions, triggers for feelings and how talking may be therapeutic. Others, though, may struggle to find words to describe their psychological state or situation, and then metaphor may help with communication and understanding.

Sometimes, people introduce their own metaphor, and here we can continue with this, perhaps extending the metaphor and deepening the meaning.

Example – *I'm in the swamp. Everywhere I stand, it's just swamp everywhere.*

We might say – *Let's think how we could start building a boardwalk across the swamp, to help keep your feet dry whilst you move to firmer ground.*

Some people may seem to us to be particularly in touch with their own creativity, describing their problems using rich, descriptive language. They may well benefit from an equally enriched therapeutic approach using metaphor.

Sometimes, we ourselves may feel that a metaphor is the easiest way to communicate an idea or treatment, perhaps to offer someone a way to manage overwhelming feelings or worries that won't go away.

Example – perhaps someone is terminally ill from cancer.

We might say – *I can't take these worries away from you, but this may perhaps help. Can you think of a piece of furniture, specifically a chest of drawers? Maybe one you own or one you remember from when you were younger, in your own house or someone else's? Now imagine opening one of the drawers – feel the handle and hear the sound whilst the drawer is opening. Now imagine putting your worries in there and tucking them all inside so they don't spill out, and slide the drawer closed. Now lock it with a key and feel the key turning in the lock. When you go out of the room, away from the chest of drawers, remember that although the worries are there, they are locked away in the drawer. You can go back in the room and open the drawer with the key anytime you like, but you can choose when you do this.*

Visual, auditory or kinaesthetic?

We can match a metaphor to a person's predominant modality for perceiving the world and how they take in and process information. We all use a combination of ways, but most of us have one that we subconsciously prefer over the others:

*   **Visual** – what we see.
*   **Auditory** – what we hear, conversations we have.
*   **Kinaesthetic** – things we touch and emotions we feel.

How do we recognise someone's preferred representational system?

Perhaps the easiest way is by listening really carefully to their language. Are there more "seeing" words, "hearing/conversation" words or "touching/feeling" words? We can then use a metaphor that aligns with their preferred system. For example, a person who uses a lot of auditory language (hearing/saying) tells us,

> *My family don't think I hear them. They disagree, but it sounds to me like I can't say anything right.*

We would choose a metaphor that uses auditory language,

> *For you, it is like **listening to a stuck record**. It **sounds** like you would prefer a **different record to play** sometimes. I wonder if there is a way for*

*you to **hear** a more positive message? Perhaps if not from the **words**, through their **tone**, or perhaps they are wanting to show they care for you and how important you are to them by **talking about you?***

Different types of metaphors and how we may use them in conversations

1 Invisible metaphors.

> Sometimes, we may use a metaphor in our head, mainly to help us, and we don't bring it into the conversation.

2 Brief metaphors/extended metaphor.

3 Specific use to help in mental health conversations to explain:

- Physiology.
- Psychological concepts.
- Medication and non-medication options.
- Prognosis.

Invisible metaphors

The following are two metaphors that we refer to as invisible, as they remain in our brain, assisting us with navigating the conversation, but usually without us actually discussing the metaphor.

Weighing scales

In some conversations, imagining a set of scales may be helpful. As someone tells their story, we listen out for the perceived problems and the perceived ability to cope and place these on each side of the scales.

Imagine a set of scales and weigh up this story,

> *I'm tired all the time and stressed... I don't know if it's because I'm not sleeping. It is not right for my children to see me like this. I have to literally drag myself from bed to do their lunchboxes and get them to school and then try and work when all I want to do is just lie in bed.*

PROBLEMS	COPING TOOLS
Tiredness, poor sleep	Routine, e.g. preparing children for school
Low motivation	Work
Feeling guilty	Love for children

Sometimes, we might share these lists, we may use hand gestures to indicate each side of the scale and present some of the main points we have heard, non-judgementally saying,

On the one hand, you are stressed about not sleeping well and struggling to do everything. On the other hand, you are managing to do the things you need to do. I think that may show how important your children are to you and how much you love them. When there is more stress, we may need more potential solutions to balance that stress.

Do you think there is a balance just now between things that feel difficult and other things that balance that? If something else was going to be added, what do you think that could be?

An onion

A second invisible metaphor that might help us to decide where to guide a conversation is considering the layers of an onion and whether we:

- Stay in the current layer and continue to explore.
- Move to an inner or outer layer.

The following is an example of using the idea of an onion with someone who tells us their mood has been low over the last few weeks.

Outer layer

Here, we may explore an overview of the person and the breadth of their situation to understand the context of their low mood, using fact-gathering questions,

What has been happening over the last few weeks?

What were things like before this?

Have you felt like this in the past? What helped then?

A layer deeper

Here, we might ask deeper questions that need more consideration than providing facts,

How is this low mood affecting your life?

Who else knows you are feeling like this? How do they know?

What do you do to cope?

Inside layer

If we move to a layer deeper again, we may encounter the emotion or information few people know about, concealed by the outer protective layers. We may build rapport before asking,

What is the most important thing to you in life right now?

What is scaring you most about this situation?

What is your biggest worry for the future?

Do you think there have been events in the past that are relevant to how you are feeling?

In this layer, we may find emotions become visible, and we may use reflection and verbal or non-verbal prompts,

I see this is bringing up a lot of emotion right now – whilst we pass a tissue.

… or give verbal permission,

It is OK to cry.

Giving permission and enabling an emotional release, such as crying, is called a cathartic encounter.

We may also think about the onion metaphor when it is clear that someone has a lot to share with us,

Are we the best person to listen? What can we do today?

Are we the best person, perhaps over a period of weeks, to peel back the onion layers?

Do we have the skills to deal with what may be there?

Sometimes, we may suspect that there is trauma, such as childhood abuse, or someone has a lot to share, and we may decide the best thing we can do is to listen. At other times, we may decide the best thing we can do is problem-solve together to determine who can be in the team of people who can listen. This may be friends, family or trained professionals.

In some situations, the worst possible thing we can do is to cut deep into the onion with a sharp knife, mainly for our own curiosity about what may be there. If we lack the skills, time or ability to deal with what we find, we may leave the person, metaphorically, weeping from the cuts. Peeling onions can end in tears.

Brief or extended metaphor

Sometimes, we may use a metaphor very briefly; at other times, we may extend it and develop a shared understanding.

Brief metaphor

An example of this is to offer a person a **magic wand**. We can use this to get an idea of what is most important to someone by asking how they would ideally like things to be; it can be a way to find out about a person's values,

*If you had a **magic wand**, what would be different for you the rest of today?*

And what would be different in your life tomorrow?

We might also use a magic wand to explain that we, as clinicians, have limited options or that our suggested treatment might take time to work,

*If I had a **magic wand**, I could give you a tablet that meant you felt instantly better today. Unfortunately, it takes at least a couple of weeks before we will know the effect of these tablets.*

Brief metaphor that we may extend

A metaphor using an **elastic band** to indicate stress can be introduced briefly or then extended to mean a shared understanding exists and to start to move to discuss management options,

*It's as if you are an **elastic band** and it has been stretched and stretched some more, until now everything feels very tense. It sounds like you are worried about what will happen if that **strained elastic band** is stretched even more. Perhaps we need to think of some ways to release some of this stretch and strain. When is a time recently that you have noticed, perhaps even briefly, the elastic band feeling even a tiny bit less stretched?*

We may extend the metaphor, providing a new way to view the situation and management,

> *Talking about this today has been an important step. I hear that life has been a struggle and that the elastic band has been stretched already, and you are looking at more stretch and strain in the future.*

> *But stretching the band could be creating resilience – the more it can stretch, the stronger it becomes – and you are a strong person. You have kept going through many challenges recently and talked about some big situations and feelings today. I think this has been an important step.*

A metaphor may be used once to share understanding of a situation, or it can be developed, as in the example below taken from ACT and used to explain the role of the clinician.

> *I am sure it feels at times like you would like to find a way to the top of the path without this struggle, perhaps a person to carry you on their shoulders.*

> *It can be disappointing and frustrating to be looking for someone to carry you and be told that all we can do is walk the path together. But we can see which path will suit you best, which tools will help and who will be most useful to accompany you on this journey.*

Specific situations

Let's consider some specific metaphors we might use to help in common mental health conversations.

Physiology

Sometimes, we need to explain a physiological process and may use a metaphor to help. At times, we would only use the metaphor. At other times, we would then add the physiology, aiming to give enough explanation for someone to understand without being overwhelmed.

Example – racing heart and anxiety.
Metaphor – primitive brain – security team,

> *Our primitive, or primal, brain is in charge of security and survival. It looks for threats and dangers and, if there is any uncertainty, it is safer for it to think the*

worst and decide there is danger. In the past, it was better for our ancestors to assume that a moving shadow was a lion rather than a tree branch, and we have inherited the same ability to scan for danger. With the security team activated, we feel on edge; unable to relax and ready to defend ourselves.

Example – racing heart, explanation of sympathetic and parasympathetic systems.

Metaphor – accelerator and brake,

When you notice your heart speeding up and thoughts racing, it is like your body's accelerator is pushed to its limit. This is your sympathetic nervous system's "fight–flight" response firing.

That needs to be counterbalanced by the brake, which is our parasympathetic nervous system or "relax–rest–digest".

Example – hyperventilation.

Metaphor – cup of tea,

When you drink a cup of tea, do you take little sips from the top and, after each sip, top up the cup?

Sometimes, without realising, we start breathing like this, taking small shallow breaths that leave most of our lungs unused, meaning we need to breathe many more times to have the same effect as one big breath.

We need to remind ourselves – particularly at times of stress – to remember the whole cup of tea and take breaths that use our diaphragm to fully empty and fill our lungs.

Psychological concepts and tools

As well as helping to explain physiological effects, we can use metaphors to help make psychological concepts clearer.

Example – brain's negative bias.

Metaphor – pin versus pencil,

Our brain is designed to be attracted to negatives. If something has not gone well or we've received negative feedback, our brain gets out a big set of pins and secures the information to the top of the noticeboard in our brain, so we remember it and keep noticing it.

On the other hand, if someone gives us a positive comment or things go the way we want, we may notice it and write it down, but this soon gets rubbed off or we pin something negative over the top, blocking our view of the positives. It can mean the only things we see are negatives.

This is the reality of what we see, but it's not the actual reality. To see more clearly, we need to consciously seek out the positives, look at them and force our brain to give these the same or greater priority.

Can you think of a way you could do this today to start getting your brain to take notice of the positives that are there and have become hidden?

Example – neuroplasticity.

Metaphor – brain muscle,

Let's imagine your brain is like a muscle. All this anxiety and worry lately is like a workout for your "worry muscle". Each time we think about a concern or feel nervous, we train the "worry muscle" to get stronger, kick in more quickly and with a bigger and faster response that can last longer.

It's like pumping our biceps and forgetting to balance it with working the triceps. The opposing muscle is really important for balance.

We need to consciously find ways to work out a "relax muscle" to train it as much as the "worry muscle". For example, eating healthy meals, getting enough sleep or calm time, being with people important to us and doing things we value or enjoy.

We could elaborate on this metaphor using the themes and language of other muscle training, for example regular practice, having a coach and finding the environment or equipment needed. Also, doing exercises several times each day, every day, will give a different outcome to just doing them once a week at the gym. We could use the example of an athlete or sportsman training for an event in the future. They would practise their skills every day in order to ensure that they are in optimum condition and as strong and fit as possible for that future event. In the same way, we can practise skills to help us manage mental health symptoms, problems or situations that we know may arise in the future. We do this when we are well, in anticipation of what will happen and not waiting for the actual moment. In this way, we have a skill set that is honed and ready to use.

We may then add an explanation of neuroplasticity,

> *Neuroplasticity is our brain's ability to rewire itself and build new neural pathways based on our behaviours, thoughts and experiences. That means we can practise, put in the time and train our brains to get better at relaxing and feeling calm.*

Example – managing thoughts or feelings.
Metaphor – driving at night,

> *Imagine we are driving at night on a dark road and we see another car coming towards us. If we focus our attention on this other vehicle, on how we are annoyed it showed up when we were enjoying our drive, we might feel angry, we might keep looking at those lights, perhaps driving towards them, making it harder to stay safely on the road.*

> *On the other hand, if we keep our eyes ahead on our lane – thinking about where we want to be going – even if it is more difficult with the other car passing, we can still stay safe and focused on our journey.*

This example can be used to discuss a person's values: what is important to them and areas to focus on and move towards. It could be used to consider what might happen: who or what (feelings, people, thoughts) might come up and be troublesome and affect us, like another car driving towards us at night.

Medications and non-medication options

Example – medication and non-medication options.
Metaphor – a rowing boat,

> *You asked about the role of medication. We could think about it like a **rowing boat**. Sometimes, the boat glides effortlessly through water. At other times, it might get stuck in the reeds or the mud. At those times, we need to think about the oars that might help get us going again.*

> *We might need different oars, all pulling together. When we feel low, the oars may be people to support us, physical activity, perhaps a way to be creative, a meaningful activity (work, caring or volunteering) and types of counselling or therapy like CBT. Medication is also an oar. We know it is more likely to be helpful when a boat is so stuck that trying other oars has not helped, and perhaps we need to use all possible oars, including medication.*

Prognosis

Example – prognosis.

Metaphor – a tree,

It is normal for us to worry about things getting worse. It is like a tree being blown around in the wind, wondering if a bigger storm is coming. Might it be enough to bring the tree down? We can start thinking about different ways in which the storm could increase.

However, it can be useful to think about the roots – these go much deeper than we have realised: self-care, activity, people who care for us and keep us anchored. We cannot know what weather will come, but we can prepare for the storm by deepening those roots and making it most likely the tree can survive. And the more the wind blows, the more the tree is stimulated to put down really deep roots so that it stays safe and anchored to the ground.

Key points – metaphors

Metaphors can help improve communication and may have therapeutic benefits, through transforming the way we see ourselves, others or the world.

They can be used in a variety of situations to share information, understanding or how a management plan will look.

Listen out and, where possible, make use of any metaphors a person introduces.

Metaphors are an opportunity for you to bring your own imagination and creativity into your conversations.

Mental health consultations in primary care

Section introduction

In this section, we will consider how to use the tools we have already described and introduce new ones. We describe common situations that we encounter in primary care:

- Anxiety and stress.
- Low mood and depression.
- Young people and older adults.
- Coping strategies that may cause problems, such as use of alcohol.
- Conversations when there is not much time.
- Conversations when there is a context of trauma.
- Working with and helping our colleagues in primary care, who may be experiencing mental health challenges.

We illustrate each chapter with three different cases. For each case, we start with the name and age of the patient and their presenting problem, with the opening line that starts the conversation. Then we explore how to manage the various challenges each case presents. Section 2 concludes by considering mental health conversations with colleagues.

DOI: 10.1201/9781003409168-8

The main tools are listed at the start of each chapter. You may spot other tools being mentioned overtly or used without specific mention; however, this list gives the main learning points or focus.

Each chapter starts with the words of a person with lived expertise in symptoms, diagnoses and health care. We find these words provide a perspective that may differ from our own. We are extremely grateful to the people who shared these. Some of these have the name of the person speaking them included, with their preference of first name or full name. Others (indicated by *) are authentic quotes but may be amalgamated from a number of people and used with an anonymised name.

6

Anxiety and stress

The voices always seemed to bother health professionals, more than they bothered me. It was with the support of the primary care team, and my partner, that I started to work on my anxiety. Being able to leave the house, get to the mail box. That is how my life started to improve.

Debra Lampshire

Introduction

The feeling of anxiety is a universal human emotion – a sense of unease, worry or fear that, at times, is entirely appropriate and may even protect us from danger. When the feeling of anxiety is strong, persistent or greater than the ability we feel we have to cope, it can become a problem and affect our well-being.

Stress is another universal experience. It is a reaction to pressure that could be physical, emotional or situational. Stress may give us motivation and energy, but it becomes a problem when it increases above a level that we feel we have the ability to manage. Stress can cause mental health problems and make existing ones worse.

Stress or anxiety can present overtly to the GP, *I am stressed*, and may be present in one or many parts of life, including work, financial, family and social. At other times, underlying stress may be less obvious, for example multiple presentations with minor illness or pain. Stress and anxiety occur on a continuum from a typical, manageable experience to one that is debilitating with huge impacts on everyday life.

DOI: 10.1201/9781003409168-9

Stress and anxiety have intertwined relationships with physical health through mechanisms such as physiological changes (e.g. increased cortisol) and neuroplasticity (e.g. structural brain changes caused by prolonged stress or anxiety).

In this chapter, we apply practical tools to three common primary care presentations involving stress and anxiety:

Example 1 – George Taylor, 45 years. Stress associated with a physical health problem.
Example 2 – Pam Littleton, 52 years. Situational anxiety.
Example 3 – Aisha Anwar, 17 years. Generalised anxiety.

Tools in this chapter

1   Coping questions.
2   Activity ladder.
3   Think, feel, do (body and you).

Additional tool

*   Image or metaphor – see Chapter 5.

Coping questions

Using coping questions enables us to find out someone's current strategies. We can hear what they are currently doing, and we might build on these in our clinical management. They make a useful assumption that the person **is** coping.

We may ask,

> *With all these stressful things going on, what are you doing that is helping you to cope?*

Activity ladder

This is a way of approaching anxiety-provoking situations or activities. We might identify these by noticing avoidance, e.g. *Oh, I don't go there anymore.* This approach offers a way to gradually build up to restart a desired activity. This is achieved by practising negotiated, manageable actions, like climbing the rungs of a ladder.

How is a step decided? We might be tempted, and think that the conversation may be quicker, if we provide the action for the next step. However, we do not know how difficult any action may be for different people at different times. It is better to ask someone what they think is manageable and for us to check this, either by reflecting this as an even smaller step or by asking for an "out of ten" rating, looking for an answer of seven or above to indicate this step is likely to be achievable.

Think, feel, do (body and you)

The tool "think, feel, do (body and you)" is based on a CBT 5-part model. In an identified situation, we consider each of these components and their interconnections. The components are:

- What we think.
- What we feel.
- What we do. This is divided into what our body does by itself, e.g. heart racing or sweating, and what actions we take, e.g. leaving the room.

Example 1 – stress associated with a physical health problem

In this case, we use coping questions and a metaphor. With these tools, we move from the start of a mental health conversation to having a next-step plan. This case demonstrates how to use these tools with someone whose own focus is on the physical pain.

Tools

- Coping questions.
- Image or metaphor – oars.

Patient	George Taylor, 45 years, male. An infrequent attender.
Past medical history (PMH)	Seen twice in the last five years, once with viral symptoms and once five weeks ago with a back injury following some home maintenance. BP 130/80. Routine bloods normal.
Social history	Works as an office manager. No children.
Opening statement	*It's my back again, it's stressing me out. Usually, I bounce straight back from anything like this. There must be something wrong.*

What do you say now?

Background

We start by asking George about his back pain. We discover bilateral lower backache currently 1–2/10 severity, present less than 20% of waking hours. There has been a gradual improvement over the last five weeks. No red flag symptoms. Back examination is normal.

Ideas	*Something is stopping me from recovering, I need to know what.*
Concerns	*The pain is another thing I don't need right now. It's a distraction at work. Work needs 100% of my focus.*
Impact	Able to undertake all normal activities. Sleep is impaired by thoughts about the pain rather than pain. Feels stressed.

We discuss pain relief and find that George's regular analgesia, given at the last consultation, is effective and there are no side effects. We wonder why George has come in, but we have noted cues,

I'm stressed out with this.

It's a distraction at work.

It's taking too long, it's not like me.

Coping questions

We decide that our first task is to zoom out to have a broader conversation beyond the physical back pain. We choose a holistic, open question,

How has everyday life been going over the last few weeks with this back pain? Which everyday activities have been different or difficult recently?

George tells us that long hours at work are "a bit of a nightmare" and have resulted in less free time and eating more takeaways. Having discovered some differences in life with the physical back pain, difficulties at work, reduced leisure time and less healthy diet, we have the opportunity to ask a coping question,

That sounds full on. It sounds as if your back is, at times, distracting you at work and also that work has been more stressful recently. I wonder if it is all interlinked, as the stress is affecting your physical health, such as eating less healthily. Also, we know that stress can mean we notice pain more. How have you been coping?

Typically, the answer to this question may not give us what we are looking for. George responds with, *Yes, things are tough. You are right, it is hard to cope.* As is often the case, we need to ask twice, and we follow up by re-asking a coping question,

> *Hmm, it does sound tough. What do you think are the things that are helping you cope?*

George answers but is still focusing on ways that he is not coping. He tells us that he has started re-checking his work and stays late to do this. This means he gets home late and has less time with his partner, who, in turn, doesn't like his work affecting their relationship.

We know that our brains have a tendency to focus on the negatives and this will happen more when we are under stress. We reflect and keep up our hunt for George's coping strategies with another similar question,

> *Compared with before, you are questioning yourself more and feel less certain in your decisions. With these current levels of stress, what do you think might be getting you through?*

George tells us that his family, particularly support from his parents and siblings, keeps him going. We ask if he does anything else, and he tells us he goes into the garden at the weekends. These are the coping strategies we were wanting to identify, and it is worth reflecting back these useful connections,

> *It seems that time in the garden and making sure you still find time to be in touch with your family are important ways to balance the stress caused by work and this back pain.*

George agrees these things help. We might check expectations at this point and ask,

> *With the back pain and the stress that has come with that, coming in today, did you have any thoughts about what might be most helpful?*

Or we may pre-empt the expected answer and include it in our question,

> *It sounds like the back pain has been affecting life quite a bit. You mentioned it is gradually improving. It would be nice if we had a magic wand and could speed that up so you could leave here pain-free. As we can't do that, do you have any particular hopes for what we might be able to do today?*

George agrees that he was probably hoping for a quick cure. He is really keen to get rid of the pain. We ask him about the main way the back pain is interfering with life, and he tells us he is worried it will get worse again and cause him to be distracted and make a mistake at work. This has not happened, but he is concerned in case it could. Within the office, he is known for his thoroughness and getting things right.

An image or metaphor

We decide to reflect this, incorporating a more holistic view of health and then introduce a metaphor,

> It is often a concern wondering about the future and "what if things get worse". It also means there are two aspects to consider: there is the back pain and the worries caused by the back pain.

> Can I explain an image of how we could think about this? I will try and draw it here. Imagine a boat gliding through the water. Suddenly, there is a current pushing against the direction of the boat, and it is slower and more difficult to keep going. Things like pain and stress are like this current. Life can feel more of an effort than normal.

> At times like this, it can help to think about the oars that keep us moving and which we might be able to add in to help us cope while we have pain **and** stresses or worries caused by the pain.

We would usually introduce this metaphor after discovering some coping tools and offer these before asking George about others,

> The oars might be targeted more at the pain or more at the worries about the pain – "What if I make a mistake at work?" – or both. It sounds to me that getting in the garden and connecting with your family help you cope with the pain and worries. Maybe your partner wanting you to get home is a support too, so you don't stay too late at work.

> At times of stress, whether that stress is caused by a physical health problem or for another reason, often we are busy focusing on the problems or the stress. We can easily forget the importance of these oars and may stop some of them, but, actually, these are the things that will keep us going and are more important than ever. Other helpful oars can be having time for sleep, physical activity and healthy food.

> Hearing all of that, do you think there are things that might be good to make time for or add back in to life?

We discuss a SMART (specific, measurable, achievable, realistic, timely) plan with George around his priority of increasing physical activity. He will plan to get off the bus to work a stop earlier and walk the remaining 10 minutes, at least three times in the next week, starting tomorrow (we reduced this from his suggestion of daily, to help it to be achievable). He will speak to family twice this week and is interested in investigating martial art classes and may start to research these. We already have two specific steps and want to encourage George but emphasise that this planning is an additional "maybe". In summary, we say,

> I am interested to see what difference you notice, if any. Getting off the bus might feel like a small thing. Sometimes, a small, regular change can create a bigger difference than you might expect. Can we plan to speak again to see how this goes?

We ask George if he prefers a phone call or face-to-face follow-up, and when to schedule this. We ensure he knows about support available 24/7 in case things suddenly feel overwhelming.

Learning point – behavioural nudge

A behavioural nudge is one small action that is achievable and can be incorporated regularly into life. A focus on "doing" means the activity is action-based rather than planning or thinking. This means that a "nudge" should be tangible and specific. For example, rather than "thinking about joining a gym", a plan might be "go and look at a local gym".

The main task of the healthcare professional is to ensure the "nudge" is small enough to be achievable – to ensure that we are setting someone up for success.

Each time the nudge action is completed, our brain endorses this with a chemical release. With regular completion of this manageable action, we create a positive association and teach our brain a new habit.

Sometimes planning one achievable change together can lead to a person adding and implementing their own additional changes. At other times, when we follow up, further support or a different approach may be needed.

Example 2 – situational anxiety

In this case, we use an activity ladder incorporating the principle of "dip your toe in rather than jumping in at the deep end". This means gradual, graded exposure to a stressful or anxiety-provoking situation, rather than a total immersion (jumping in at the deep end). It is important that each exposure is small enough to be achievable. This success is built on with moving to the next rung up on the ladder.

Tool

- Activity ladder.

Telephone consultation

Patient	Pam Littleton, 52 years, female.
PMH	Recent telephone consultation with your colleague. Given fit note/off-work for two weeks for "work-related stress". Mild hypertension, well controlled on a once-daily medication. All blood tests and recent blood pressure (BP) normal.
Social history	Work – cleaner for contract cleaning company; three children (17, 18 and 19 years).
Opening statement	*I won't take up your time, I just need another week off work, can you do me a note?*

What do you say now?

Background

On the phone, we introduce ourselves and explain our role and that our colleague is away. We ask for some background information, and Pam tells us about workplace bullying by colleagues teasing, and moving things from her cleaning trolley as a joke; an HR process is underway. She does have two friends amongst her colleagues. Her teenagers are "being teenagers". She says, *I can't cope with going back.* Away from work, the last two weeks, she has felt better. We find out her ICE:

Ideas	*I can't cope at work. I need more time off.*
Concerns	*I am using up a lot of sick leave.*
Expectations	A sick note.

When we explored her concerns, we found out that she had planned to go back today and had actually gone in this morning. She was about to enter the locker room when she felt dizzy and had to leave. She returned home, where she felt better and made this appointment.

We reflect what we have heard and check we share the same understanding of the problem,

> It sounds as if, on the one hand, you are keen to go back to work even with the ongoing HR process. You do have colleagues you consider friends. Returning to work is also important from a financial point of view and, of course, not using up sick leave. On the other hand, when you went in today, it sounds as if you experienced a strong and immediate reaction with dizziness and the feeling that you had to get out.

Information giving

We include some explanation around our fight–flight response,

> Our brain's job is to keep us safe, detecting danger or potential dangers and then putting us into our "high alert" or "fight/flight" state. When you went to open the locker room today, it sounds as if your brain identified a potential danger – which is understandable given your experiences.

> However, feeling dizzy, probably from breathing faster, and the thought, "I need to get out of here" – although your brain was trying to keep you safe – got in the way of what you wanted, which was to work.

Activity ladder

We next introduce the idea of an activity ladder,

> Can I explain what I think happened? There has been stress and anxiety with the situation at work. It is good that you have felt more relaxed during the time away. In order to return to work now, we need to ease back into it, like the saying "dip your toe in, rather than jumping in at the deep end". I would say that going straight back into work today, and the reaction you experienced, was like jumping in at the deep end.

Next, we ask Pam for suggestions to set up a ladder of activity,

> If going in to work today was like jumping in at the deep end, what would be something that would be a smaller step, like dipping your toe in...? Something towards going to work, but that feels manageable...?

Pam suggests going in for half a shift. We want to hold this answer up to the "truth light". How would this be different from this morning? Would it be manageable enough to be achieved? Can we start with something even smaller? If needed, we could use a 1–10 scale to determine how stressful this would feel. We ask Pam what would be a first step up the ladder. Pam suggests putting her uniform on at home, as she felt a bit nervous when she was packing it to bring to work.

We may work through one or two of the first rungs of the ladder and leave this as a "behavioural nudge" recognising that Pam may add more to herself. As a reminder, a behavioural nudge is an action that a person can take towards the goal, aiming to set up for success. Depending on the situation and person, you may decide to complete just one step on the ladder and then check in again later.

We might also include a relaxation strategy in this conversation,

If you try this first step of putting on your uniform at home and experience similar feelings to today or other signs of being in "high alert" mode, is there something else you could do at the same time? Something to balance those feelings and try to give a calmer, relaxed message to your brain?

If we need to offer suggestions, we may add,

Some people find they will take a deep breath or think of a place or person that makes them feel calm, chew gum or sip a drink. Different options will work best for different people. What do you think you would try?

We discuss Pam's idea of listening to relaxing music. She often wears headphones at work, so this would be something she could also use later on other steps of the ladder.

Specific conversational tool – activity ladder

The activity ladder is a form of graded exposure. It can be used for anxiety related to a certain place or event, e.g. the workplace, or a particular assessment or exam.

Think of a ladder where the top rung is the situation or activity causing anxiety. We start by standing and looking at the ladder. Our role is to describe the plan and to make the steps – particularly the first – small enough, and then make it smaller again to ensure a successful start.

(Continued)

Once the first step has been taken and practised, we can look to the next rung.

A crucial part of the role of the healthcare professional is to check whether a step is small enough to be achievable. If not, then we can help with breaking the step down further.

There can be strong urges to avoid or stop taking a step. As well as making this small and then smaller and practising as we go, other strategies can be added to balance the potential stress. This might be with something the person finds calming, perhaps listening to music or chewing gum.

Example 3 – generalised anxiety

Tool

- Think, feel, do (body and you).

This is an example of a "zoom-in" conversation, where we focus on one particular feeling or situation and discuss this in detail.

Typically, this conversation is based on a previous specific experience, but it can be used in a generalised way by encompassing past and present. The difference between these would be:

Past – *When you were at the supermarket and noticed your heart racing, what thoughts went through your head?*

... compared with:

Present – *At times when you feel anxious and notice your heart racing, what thoughts go through your mind?*

Patient	Aisha Anwar, 17 years, female.
PMH	None. No allergies or medications.
Social history	Lives with parents and siblings. Eldest of three.
Opening statement	*Mum said I should come in; my anxiety is getting worse.*

What do you say now?

Background

Aisha tells us that she has come in because of "worse anxiety". We discover that she has not been going out to spend time with her friends. Her mum is concerned, as she is quieter around the house and spends a lot of time in her bedroom. She has started checking the electric plug sockets around the house before she can get to sleep. This caused an argument this morning after her dad and brother discovered their mobile phones were not charged. We listen and hear her ICE:

Ideas	*I am anxious and it's interfering with my life.*
Concerns	*It is getting worse.*
Expectation	*I need a plan.*

Think, feel, do (body and you)

First, we identify a situation,

> *Can you think of a time recently when you noticed feeling "worse anxiety"?*

Aisha identifies this morning when her brother and dad were annoyed. We confirm some details. This took place in the kitchen where Aisha had prepared her breakfast. We start with an open question inviting a response from any of thinking, feeling or doing,

> *What did you notice happening when you were in the kitchen and noticed "worse anxiety"?*

If we need to direct the discussion, we might add a second question,

> *Maybe a thought or worry or something in your body like your heart racing?*

Aisha tells us her mind is blank, and she can't think clearly, but she did notice her heart racing and worried it might get faster or she might have a heart attack. Different people will notice different aspects of think, feel, do, and some of these will be easier for them to express than others. We reflect what she noticed and explore,

> *At times like this, it sounds as if there is a lot happening in your body, with your heart racing in a way you can't ignore. Do you notice other changes?*

Aisha feels like she might vomit. We explore the thoughts and worries she had this morning,

> *When you were in this situation with the argument over the phones not having charged, your body responded with nausea and heart racing. When your heart was racing, you had some worrying thoughts, such as "What if I have a heart attack?" What other worries were going through your mind?*

Aisha tells us she doesn't understand why this happened because usually her anxiety only affects her when she is in a big group of people. We reflect,

> *Sounds like you were thinking, "Why is this happening now, at home?" How did that make you feel?*

Aisha tells us she was worried that she would be late for school and have to get a bus without her friends, and her teacher would shame her in front of the class for arriving late. We could reflect these thoughts before asking again about feelings,

> *You started thinking – "I might miss my usual bus". "I might be late for school". How did that feel?*

Aisha says she felt annoyed with her brother. Finally, we ask what she did,

> *If your family were watching you closely while all this was happening, what would they have seen you doing?*

She tells us that she sat still, and couldn't eat her breakfast. Now, we have information for each part of the model.

Whilst having the conversation, we have made connections. We may choose to summarise and emphasise these connections,

> *Let's think about the situation this morning when you noticed "worse anxiety". We could break this down into parts. It sounds, perhaps, as if the first change you noted in your body was your heart beating faster. You had thoughts: "I might have a heart attack" and "What if I miss the bus?" Those are worrying thoughts, which could speed up your heart rate. You sat there and were unable to eat your breakfast.*

What can we do now?

We could decide to continue the conversation with one of the following four options:

1 Add to the model.
2 Introduce a metaphor.
3 Plan a change.
4 Zoom out.

Let's explore each of these.

Add to the model

Often, someone will find some parts of the model easier to notice and discuss than others. One next step, particularly if one of the parts has much less content than others, may be to suggest someone consider these aspects in a different situation,

> *Perhaps, in a different situation, you may notice some of these same "what if" worries, or nausea and heart racing, or you may notice different or extra things. This will be useful for us to understand this feeling of anxiety better.*

We may suggest Aisha thinks about or writes these down. If we have already written down the information she has shared, we could give this to her so she can add to it. This can be considered a form of personalised psycho-education or getting to know yourself. See diagram on page 57.

This may be a good point to end this part of the conversation with the suggestion that she thinks about each of these components (think, feel and do) in further situations.

Metaphor – snowball

We may want to use a metaphor to emphasise the connections between the parts of the model and why this understanding is helpful,

> *Can you imagine a snowball rolling down a mountain? It gets bigger and faster as it goes. Anxiety can feel like this. We feel caught up, and the thinking-feeling-doing may feel as if it is getting bigger and more out of control. The thought: "Should I call an ambulance?" can trigger our heart to race and us to fidget and feel anxious. The sensation of heart racing reinforces the thought that perhaps we may need an ambulance.*

We can use this metaphor to introduce the idea of trying to change one of the parts to see what effect it could have overall,

> *All the thinking, feeling and doing that we were talking about are wrapped up in that snowball. If we change just one of these – even a little bit – it can change the inevitable course of rolling faster and growing bigger. The more we can start to notice and understand the very first signs when the snowball is still small, the easier it can be to change. This could make a bigger, quicker difference. So, understanding those first thoughts, feelings and what your body and you are doing can be helpful.*

Planning for change

We might discuss options for change. Focusing on behaviour, we would start by asking about something that could be done differently,

> *Now that we have discussed how these are connected, we can try changing one thing, for example what you were doing, to see if it makes a difference to other connected things, like how anxious you were feeling. This morning when you felt "worse anxiety" you said you were sitting very still. What could you try doing differently, in a similar situation?*

Zoom out

So far, we have zoomed in on one situation. We might decide to end with zooming out and use an overall coping question, for example a treasure hunt tool, to ask something like,

> *With experiencing worse anxiety, what things are you doing differently, or not doing, compared with how you were before?*

Using the metaphor, we might explore ways that would make the snowball less likely to start forming in the first place.

Aisha tells us that she used to spend time with her friends, going to each other's houses to study or to the shops. We discuss a specific plan to restart this – contacting a friend today and going to a friend's house within the next week, even for a short time.

Top tips for talking about anxiety and stress

Listen closely for a person's current coping strategies or strengths, and reflect these back:

- When a person says, *I just keep going,* you can reflect this back as, *Even when things are tough, you can focus on what you need to do.*

- When a person says, *I have worked there for six years,* you can reflect this back as,
  You must have knowledge, skills and expertise that someone just starting would not have.

If someone finds it difficult to address stress or a mental health problem, consider starting with interventions that benefit both physical and mental health, for example getting outdoors, increasing movement, improving sleep or diet.

Plan for success. We all like our own ideas best, so remember to ask rather than suggest. Then, discuss and agree the next step together, building on strengths and current ways of coping.

Arrange follow-up. This can help with motivation and accountability for the agreed next step. It can also increase rapport, demonstrating we are on the journey together. The follow-up conversation will help us review what has worked and what hasn't to continue or re-think the plan.

Health anxiety

> We had to wait for Dad's appointment. Then, we were told we had to wait and see a specialist. We got more and more anxious. We didn't know of any ways to deal with that.
>
> **Kat★**

Introduction

A conversation about health anxiety will often start with a physical health problem: a swelling, pain, tingling or a change somewhere in the body. This is our first focus – sometimes it might feel tempting to have physical health as the only focus. But most people with symptoms already have thoughts and worries – this is why we are taught to ask about ideas, concerns and expectations. Sometimes the anxiety about the physical symptom is significant and is stopping someone from living their life in the way they want. It is important that we explore worries about physical symptoms to identify when this is the case.

Some physical symptoms, perhaps palpitations or bowel changes at times of stress, will make us wonder if anxiety may be a cause. Although we may wish to discuss anxiety, we may be unsure how to introduce this change in focus.

If someone asks for help with feeling low or anxious, there is instantly a shared agreement on the problem focus. With health anxiety, we may need additional tools to shift the conversation to the worrying thoughts.

How can I guide a conversation beyond the physical symptom(s)?

Here are some transition questions. We may use two or three, often focused on ideas and concerns – thoughts and worries.

We could start with an open question,

> *What thoughts have you had about...?*

Then,

> *What worries you about...?*

If necessary, we can normalise,

> *If this were me, my brain would be worrying about many things – perhaps, "What's causing this?" or "What might happen next?" What's gone through your mind?*

If we need to ask more, we can ask,

> *What are the most worrying thoughts you have had about this?*

> *When your brain starts to really worry, what does it come up with?*

> *Do you have other worries about your health aside from this lump?*

> *Are you also worrying about other things in your life?*

A good time to ask these questions may be when there is less eye contact and less direct focus on the conversation. When our attention is apparently diverted elsewhere, it can be easier for us to ask these questions in a way that sounds casual and may therefore be easier to answer. For example:

- In a face-to-face conversation when standing to start or finish a physical examination.
- In a video or phone call, signposting that you are looking at the computer to review or type up notes.

"Thoughts" may be an easier starting point than "worries".

Is anxiety relevant when someone has physical symptoms?

When someone has multiple physical symptoms, we may well consider the role of anxiety; remember that when we practise worrying, we get good at it and naturally do it more.

But shouldn't I deal with the physical symptoms first?

Of course, it is essential to be a safe clinician and to always have in mind that any symptoms may well have a significant physical cause – something that we need to find out, diagnose and treat in order to be safe and best help the patient. However, let's imagine for a moment that the physical symptoms are in a basket, at the bottom of a cliff below, out of sight but attached to a rope. Each time we learn more about the physical symptoms, imagine we pull the rope lifting the basket upwards. We won't know until the basket gets to the top, and we can see in, whether this physical problem has a purely physical answer. It can take time and several conversations to get there.

What if, when the basket reaches the top, we look inside only to find it does not have the expected content? No physical answer (diagnosis) is found for symptoms. All our effort has been focused on this physical problem and it now feels harder to introduce a new focus. Even if there is a physical answer, time with unaddressed worries has increased anxiety and adversely affected life.

Discussing thoughts and worries about the physical symptoms in each conversation, however difficult, will help us provide holistic care and ensure people are prepared, whatever the diagnosis.

Tools in this chapter

1 Detective, judge and court reporter - identify, assign and discuss.
2 Choose the focus.
3 Managing a tunnel thought.

Additional tools

* Coping questions – see Chapter 2
* Image or metaphor – see Chapter 5.

Detective, judge, court reporter

First, we identify that there are two issues – the problem and the worries about the problem. Then we assess each of these for impact.

The detective explores the first issue and then looks for the second:

1 Identify and discuss the main symptom(s) [physical].
2 Identify and discuss thoughts and worries [anxiety].

At this point, the conversations are separate.

The judge assesses the impact of each issue and assigns responsibility.

The court reporter summarises and opens a discussion.

See the box, 'Conversational tool', later in this section for more details.

Choose the focus

This tool can be helpful when one thought, emotion or physical symptom obscures a wider view of a situation. If all my focus is on feeling angry and I notice that my fists are clenched, I could shift my focus to take a slow breath, or notice what sounds I can hear inside and outside the room I am in. This widens my focus to my body and where I am. We might guide this and mirror someone who is tensing their hands doing the same with ours and saying,

I can see both our hands are clenched. Can you stretch out your fingers?

… while also stretching out ours. Or we may ask,

Can you hear that? There are often lorries going past. That sounded like one.

We might ask whether things feel any different now with this small change, or we might explain that sometimes we can zoom in so much that it can feel a relief to zoom out and notice other things as well.

Tunnel thoughts

A tunnel thought is not a tool, but is a useful cue to notice. Sometimes, we can't get a certain negative thought out of our head, or we may be in a conversation where, as much as we try to discuss other things, we keep being presented with the same statement. It is as if we are in a tunnel and the only direction is towards this one idea. Someone may repeatedly state,

> *I have left it too late to start revising.*

This could represent a **core belief**. For example, the idea *I always fail* may underpin this thought. It could indicate wider stress and anxiety that we might discover by asking about other life stresses. It is worth us noticing, reflecting and discussing a tunnel thought. We can find out whether these are getting in the way of life, or if someone has ways to cope with these thoughts. We might discuss approaches, such as "choose the focus" or, in some cases, discuss involving others such as psychological services.

Let's explore some examples:

Example 1 – Leon Jones, 23 years. Concerns about cancer.

Example 2 – Mark Masefield, 41 years. Can't catch my breath.

Example 3 – Miss Sarah Williams, MD, 39 years. Health anxiety in a health professional.

Example 1 – concerns about cancer

Here, we consider a person worried about cancer and explore ways to have a conversation about a physical symptom and health anxiety.

Tools

- Detective, judge, court reporter.
- Coping questions.

Patient	Leon Jones, 23 years, male.
PMH	Nothing of note – new patient.
Social history	Third-year university student. Keen soccer player.
Behaviour	Quiet.
Opening statement	*Is this lump on my arm cancer?*

What do you say now?

Leon has told us he has a physical lump – this could be cancer. First, we want to find out the details of the lump.

Detective

The first conversation

> *Can you tell me more about the lump? Then I will have more of an idea about what it might be and be able to answer your question.*

He first noticed the lump a couple of years ago but ignored it and then noticed it again last week. It is painless, has no effect on arm function. He is otherwise physically well.

The second conversation

> *You asked whether this could be cancer. What other thoughts, or worries, did you have about this lump?*

He tackled someone at soccer a few weeks ago and hit his arm, it could have come up after that. He is worried it could be a cancer that has spread. His best friend's dad has recently been diagnosed with cancer. One of his problems was lumps, maybe under the arm,

> *We all have times when our brains start to think worrying thoughts. What else has your brain been thinking about, for example if you are sitting quietly or lying in bed?*

Leon thinks he has the same cancer as his friend's dad. His friend has been very upset, and they are not sure how long his dad will live. He worries when he is with his friend and sometimes when he is with his family. He has no real worries about the rest of life; normal stresses of study and part-time work.

Judge

We weigh the balance; it seems that the worries are affecting his life him more than the lump itself. We explore this,

> *With this lump and these worries, are there things you are doing differently now?*

Leon has been spending more time in his room on the internet – often reading about cancer – and not seeing friends.

Court reporter

> *You came about this lump. Right now, it is not stopping you from doing anything, but you have been thinking about it and what would happen if it were cancer. These worries have affected you – spending more time alone. I wonder if we need two plans – one for the lump and one for the worries about the lump. What do you think?*

At this point, we may need further tests or opinions, or we may be able to provide reassurance and a safety plan of when to return.

Outcome 1 – further tests or opinions needed

It is hard for our brains to deal with uncertainty so while we are figuring out what is going on with this lump, shall we make a plan to manage these "what if" thoughts?

Outcome 2 – reassurance

From talking to you and examining you, I am reassured this lump is from the injury and not cancer. I expect it to go away in the next two weeks, but if not or if it changes, let's check it again. But perhaps, despite this, there will be times when you find yourself thinking again that it could be cancer or other worrying thoughts. Shall we plan what to do when you get those thoughts?

Leon agrees and we use coping questions,

Recently, what have you done when your brain gets busy with worrying thoughts?

Does it help?

Is there anything else you have tried that helps you cope with the thoughts?

Leon reflects that being alone in his room reading about cancer does not help, as it makes him worry more. Listening to music and going for a walk can help. Being around other people helps too, even if he does think of the lump.

You decide together that, after dinner, he will stay in the living room and socialise. He will go to soccer and for a walk on the other days.

Specific conversational tool – detective, judge, court reporter (identify, assign, discuss)

This tool provides a way to talk about physical and mental health symptoms together. We identify the presenting symptom and look for clues of an additional contributing factor, remembering that mental health may be a cause or consequence of the initial symptom. Then, we assess the impacts of each (typically divided into physical and mental). Next, we share and discuss this information. We can think of the stages of this conversation as taking on the roles of a detective, then a judge and then a court reporter.

(Continued)

105

The detective identifies the two conversations by exploring the first issue and then looking for the second conversation,

> *You have come in about the back pain (1), what worries you most about this?*
>
> *OK, a big worry is that you may need to give up work due to the pain (2).*

The judge notes these two areas and assesses the impact of each, to assign responsibility,

> Asking specifically, we discover that there is no pain at night but she does lie awake worrying. We decide that while back pain affects her day, the worries disturb her sleep.

The court reporter summarises and checks whether the person agrees with the approach,

> *I think we have two things going on. The back pain and then the worries the back pain is giving you about the future. I think these worries are definitely affecting your sleep and it is worth talking about both of these. What do you think?*

Example 2 – can't catch my breath

In this case, the predominant symptom is a physical sensation of shortness of breath, which has a close link with mental health. Those with respiratory diagnoses causing shortness of breath may notice anxiety linked to "not being able to get enough air". Conversely, when we see someone with shortness of breath, we need to consider anxiety as a potential cause or contributing factor.

This discussion includes a tool to use at the time of the symptom and tools for when there are no symptoms, aiming to lessen or prevent their recurrence.

Breathing problems can soon make us feel out of control, so it is useful to develop an understanding and have a plan to quickly regain control.

Tools

- Choose the focus.
- Image or metaphor – training for an event, in between events.

Patient	Mark Masefield, 41 years, male.
PMH	Hypertension, hyperlipidaemia. Muscle aches from statin.
Medication	Angiotensin receptor blocker (ARB) only. Not on statin.
Social history	Delivery driver (supermarket food orders). Non-smoker. Likes weightlifting.
Opening statement	*I can't catch my breath.*

What do you say now?

Background

We ask open questions and learn that recently, on several occasions at work, Mark has suddenly felt unable to breathe. This has come on quickly, lasting a few minutes. He has no exertional breathlessness, wheezing or cough, nocturnal snoring or apnoea, or other respiratory symptoms. There is no chest pain. The shortness of breath feels like not getting enough air, with tingling in the fingers. There are no red flags and no risk factors for asthma. You find out Mark's thoughts and worries:

Ideas – *There's something wrong with my heart or lungs.*
Concerns – *I might have to go off sick or even be unable to work.*

Your working hypothesis is anxiety.

We take the opportunity to discuss what is important to Mark and empathise. We reflect,

> It sounds like your job is important to you, and it's upsetting to think of this problem with your breathing getting in the way of being able to work. I think your employer must feel lucky to have an employee who is as dedicated to their work as you are.

Often, at this point, someone will tell us more about what's important to them. Mark has always enjoyed his work. It took a while to be accepted as part of the team, but he has now worked for the same supermarket in various roles for 17 years.

We now think it is likely that Mark, like anyone with breathing/panic or strong anxiety feelings, feels out of control when unable to catch his breath.

Sharing this can help us move the conversation to a deeper rapport and understanding. We reflect this and check in to allow Mark to tell us more,

> *Coming back to these breathing episodes, I'm hearing they come on without warning and hit you fast, almost as if you are out of control.*

Mark nods vigorously and confirms that this scares him. He tells us he gets light-headed, with tingling fingers. He tries to take deep breaths, but it gets stuck like he can't breathe. Once, in the van, he thought he really should pull over, but he was on a motorway and instead focused really hard on the road.

As Mark describes this, we notice he is taking bigger gasps, and we can see rapid rising and falling of his chest.

Choose the focus

We decide to use the tool "Choose the focus" and present this using language around being in control. We are seeking to move or expand the focus so that, **as well as** the sensation of being unable to catch his breath, he experiences being in control of his body in other ways. We say,

> *I think I would find that scary. Looking at you now, I'm wondering if you are experiencing a little of the breathing and out-of-control feeling right now. What could you do straight away to let your brain know that you are in control?*

If Mark responds to this by suggesting an option it will probably fall into one of two categories: something he can do, *I could go for a walk*, or something he could think, *I tell myself, I can get through this*. In this case, Mark does not answer and seems distracted. We suspect this is because Mark may have increasing anxiety, or the start of a panic attack, so we give a clear instruction and physical demonstration,

> *Right now, can you tense one of your hands into a fist, really tight, then stretch out your fingers, using a lot of energy to separate them as far away from each other as you can? Yes — just like that. Perhaps you were starting to feel that same out-of-control feeling, but you are in control. You are choosing to move your hand. How does your breathing feel now?*

We discuss trying this technique when Mark first notices any sign of stress; thinking, feeling or body response.

Here, we have explored an episode of dysfunctional breathing, introducing the term "feeling out of control". Then we find a way – involving an action or "doing" – to feel in some way "in control". Applying ACT theory, we are not trying to *distract* him from breathing or worrying thoughts; we are accepting that these thoughts are here and that feeling short of breath can be a normal physiological response to stress. The aim is to use an action to prompt the thought *I am in control*, and for this thought to prompt physiological change, including a slowing of the breathing.

An image or metaphor – training

We could continue this conversation and consider ways to try and prevent these episodes. Mark has told us he has taken up weightlifting and may even consider doing this competitively. We use this to provide a metaphor for "training",

> *If you were training for an event, you would have tools and techniques you would practise in advance to use on the day, during the event. Thinking about your breathing, there are some techniques that you might find will help you feel in control at the time when you notice feeling short of breath. There are also helpful training tools to practise between events at times when your breathing feels normal.*

We check in and ask Mark if he has ever tried any breathing exercises, what they were and how helpful or unhelpful he found them. Mark tells us he has heard about this sort of thing but has not done any himself other than breathing as he normally does every day! We ask whether he might have time to try some "low and slow" breathing in bed, and he says he will give it a try. We endorse this decision and describe one option for breathing,

> *I think it would be worth a try because sometimes, without realising it, we are breathing a bit faster than normal, and this can make us more likely to experience feeling short of breath. Practising deep, slow breathing each day may help. Breathe in really slowly, making sure air is going all the way to the bottom of our lungs, pushing out our lower ribs, and then breathe slowly out. Even just one minute, using five breaths can, over time, help train us back into slower breathing all the time.*

Mark decides he might be able to try this when stopped at traffic lights and one minute before sleep every day.

Top tips for talking about breathing

We may interpret yawning as indicating poor sleep, but it can be a response to hyperventilation. If someone frequently yawns, mouth breathes or uses accessory muscles, during a conversation, consider the benefits of breathing exercises.

Hyperventilation may not be an obvious fast gasping for air. Even breathing a couple of extra breaths per minute can lead to symptoms of hyperventilation. It is very common for this to be either a cause of or a physiological response to anxiety.

A quick assessment of breathing can be done by placing one hand on the chest and one on the upper abdomen: which hand moves most when breathing in? The aim is that the hand over the chest – along with the neck and shoulders – moves less or doesn't move.

To strengthen the diaphragm, we can use exercises that target this muscle. Lie on your back with hands behind your head ("beach pose"). This prevents the use of accessory muscles. Place a wheat pack or book over the upper abdomen. Notice that this item lifts when breathing in through the nose.

There are many options for breathing exercises. Prolonging the exhale phase seems particularly beneficial for mood.[1] Accompany this with an image such as floating in the sea, with each breath in carrying you up the wave to the crest and then breathing out down the wave. Take 10 breaths over two minutes out to sea and the same back. Or imagine a cat lying on the top of our stomach/lower ribs, being soothed to sleep with smooth breaths, in and out.

Example 3 – health anxiety in a health professional

Imagine your next patient is a neurosurgeon worried about a new headache. How do you feel? Conversations with our colleagues can feel daunting. As health professionals, we might notice that we would like to defer to our specialist colleague or we may want to ensure the dynamic keeps us in a position of power (see ego states in Chapters 4 and 11). The health professional patient may feel embarrassed or that they are risking losing status either by attending with something relatively trivial or, conversely, that they have neglected.

How can I talk with a patient who is a health professional?

While some of these consultations can feel the same as any other, there may be differences. We may adjust our consultation skills to fit a health professional patient better.

Hierarchy

First, let's consider ourselves. Do we notice that we change or exaggerate our conversational style with a health professional patient, particularly related to hierarchy? Do we tend to feel inferior or superior? Do we display this or overcompensate for it? Understanding how we may respond, particularly under pressure, can help us notice and then consciously return to an equal partnership.

Colleagues

Sometimes we may be tempted to interact with our professional patient as if we were colleagues, for example by discussing an educational event or asking them a professional question to save us from waiting for a formal response. A brief mention of a shared experience could be a way to build rapport; however, we need to ensure that we set up a conversation where our role is being the health professional for our colleague.

Jargon

Jargon can help identify someone as a health professional, *You mentioned 'paraesthesia'; do you work in health?* In most consultations we consciously avoid medical jargon, but does this matter with a health professional patient? Would using jargon or shared language help us to form a partnership and build rapport? Perhaps, but, in many specialities, acronyms may have different meanings and a commonly used term in one may be rarely used in another. We may balance this by using normal patient language and adding jargon that is **first** used by the health professional patient.

Ourselves

Sharing our experiences of also being a health professional and patient may help, demonstrating that we appreciate the dual roles. Our "I" statements may have particular value in validating and prompting a conversation,

> *It can be reassuring to have knowledge of different conditions, but, at other times, I think I may worry more, knowing about many potentially concerning reasons for a headache.*

Patient and professional

Within an equal partnership between a health professional and a patient who is also a health professional, there is the opportunity for unique conversations. We may choose to overtly identify these,

> *What would your thoughts be about these headaches if you were to answer in your professional role?*

Exploring ideas, concerns and expectations is invariably useful in these conversations and can give us new areas to consider, but we may need to be particularly aware of being anchored to a particular diagnosis that may be unlikely, or mean we miss the actual cause or most important aspect of a presentation.

Tunnel thoughts and health professionals

We may encounter a health professional patient who is fixed to a particular diagnosis or management. In health, we use our brains professionally to filter information and make decisions. We like to think we are doing this rationally and we trust our brain's ability to objectively interpret symptoms. This is not the case. We are all susceptible to the influence of various biases and can misinterpret our own and others' symptoms.

Additionally, regardless of professional knowledge, a thought or feeling does not equal a fact. For example:

I feel anxious (feeling) does not equal *Something bad **will** happen* (fact).
I think this stomach ache is similar to my patient who had cancer (thought) does not equal *I have cancer* (fact).

We have probably all had times when we have worried about our health based on interpreting a thought or feeling as a fact, e.g. *I keep forgetting things* (thought) = a brain tumour (fact).

Identifying a tunnel thought provides an opportunity to validate anxieties and discuss these.

How can I move a conversation from a tunnel thought?

What else have you considered?

What about a non-physical cause? What made you rule that out?

Do you think we have enough information on [these alternatives]?

How is this thought affecting you day-to-day?

Who else have you spoken to about this?

If you discussed this as a case with your colleagues, what ideas might they suggest?

If you were completing or writing this as an exam case, what would the most likely answer be?

In the following example, we talk with a worried health professional, using some of the tools outlined earlier.

Tools

- Identifying and managing tunnel thoughts.
- Coping questions.

Patient	Miss Sarah Williams, 39 years, female.
PMH	Six months – intermittent upper abdominal pain. Ultrasound scan and computerised tomography (CT) scan of abdomen and pelvis normal. Full set of blood tests all normal
Social history	Consultant general surgeon, local hospital. Single.
Behaviour	Anxious/embarrassed.
Opening statement	*This intermittent pain in the epigastrium is ongoing and imaging has not shown anything. I really need an answer to what is causing it.*

What do you say now?

Background

We hear the anxiety in her voice and note she uses medical jargon rather than words most patients would use. We review the details of the pain: it is intermittent with no triggers, lasting up to 60 minutes. There are no associated features except for occasional nausea, and no other gastrointestinal, bladder, gynaecological symptoms, or possibility of pregnancy. The pain has been unchanged since previous reviews and imaging. We find out Sarah's ICE:

Ideas –	*Pain not going, there must be something wrong.*
Concerns –	*It might be a rare cancer. Someone in the team mentioned a patient – a woman in her 30s with a rare pancreatic cancer who presented initially with vague abdominal symptoms. An early scan would have picked this up.*
Expectations –	A prompt referral for a magnetic resonance imaging (MRI) scan and second opinion.

We are wondering whether Sarah has a "tunnel thought" and decide to check this out by asking about her experience so far,

> *Wearing your health professional hat, what other thoughts have you had about what this could be? Sitting here now, which of these possibilities worries you most?*

> *Right now, for you, which feels most likely?*

We notice that Sarah seems to have this rare condition as a tunnel thought, coming back to it in her answer to each of these questions. With these answers, normal investigations and unchanged symptoms, we decide to use this tunnel thought as a cue and take the lead on introducing the role of anxiety,

> *When thinking broadly about causes of abdominal pain, I would have anxiety somewhere on the list.*

Sarah has not considered this and thinks it unlikely. We decide to introduce the idea of anxiety as a consequence of the pain, rather than a cause,

> *Right now, there is a thought that this pain could be caused by an early, rare pancreatic cancer but there is uncertainty. We do not know that it is cancer; the tests so far have not shown that, but the question is still there. This uncertainty can be difficult. Some people will say that not knowing is more stressful than receiving a diagnosis and starting some form of treatment. How are you coping with this current uncertainty?*

Sarah acknowledges that it feels difficult. She feels alone in trying to find out what is going on – that people just want to reassure her. We ask about this "feeling alone" by repeating Sarah's words,

> *That is a difficult position, feeling you are the only one who is fighting to find out the cause of the pain. Do you mean feeling alone when you are the patient in a consultation or at other times?*

Sarah says it is a bit of both. We ask about other healthcare encounters: Sarah has not had issues as a patient but remains concerned that the pain is caused by cancer. We ask how things are at work and hear that there have been some departmental changes. A close colleague has left and there is a new head of department, causing some stress. When we ask Sarah about who might support her outside work, she tells us she would not readily talk to others about her own health issues. If there was a real problem, she might involve her parents. We validate this saying,

I think as health professionals we may sometimes feel that, with our own health, we should continue to take a lead role, as at work, and manage alone. Sometimes this works, but at other times it might prevent us from getting useful support. If you were going to speak to someone else about this today, maybe about the pain and/or the stress at work, who would that be? Your parents? Or someone else?

Sarah has a friend, they don't usually talk about this sort of thing but, without a diagnosis, she would not want to bother her parents and would speak to this friend. They had mentioned meeting up soon. This has given us a coping strategy. We decide to add another coping strategy and ask,

With the uncertainty about the cause of the pain, recent changes at work and no doubt many day-to-day work challenges, what helps you cope?

Sarah likes hill walking and getting out in nature but hasn't done this in a while. Having built some rapport and understood more of Sarah's context, we decide to return to the tunnel thought and Sarah's request for a referral for an MRI. We decide to ask further about her coping strategy of having more investigations and how well this has reassured her so far,

You were hoping for answers and reassurance from the ultrasound and CT scan. Would you agree? Did it work? Were you reassured? How long did that feeling last? What do you expect to happen with an MRI? Do you think there is any chance, however small, that the MRI result could be the same as the other tests? Sometimes knowing a result is reassuring does not mean we feel reassured.

We might summarise further and explain our own role,

On the one hand we have these normal tests. There are limits to any test, as you have said, but, overall, it is very reassuring that no cancer has been found. On the other hand, you are still wondering whether this pain is being caused by pancreatic cancer. It is normal to want an answer. Using our medical brains, we would think about adding investigations, and that an MRI is the best next step. It is an interesting conundrum that we can know a scan is normal and yet still feel anxious. Part of my role is to work out what we want; in this case, an answer – fully excluding pancreatic cancer and reassurance – and the best way to get to this.

While holding our role as the health professional, we open a conversation about a trial period of managing anxiety without the scan,

The investigations we have so far are reassuring. I am interested to know if any features of the pain may change with a focus on managing the stress linked

with the uncertainty. It may change in a way that makes it easier for us to understand the cause or it might not make any difference. I wonder how you would feel about trying the plan to restart some regular hill walking and get in touch with your friend. Let's monitor any changes and meet again soon. We can talk more then about an MRI or other investigations.

At the next consultation we again talk about the pain. We also want to find out any other worries that might have been hiding behind this and ask a general question – whether she has concerns about any other areas of her life. Sarah has been thinking about the patient with the rare cancer: she remembers being struck by the fact that this patient was trying for a pregnancy. This is something she puts off thinking about, but that causes her distress. She had considered freezing her eggs but became busy and now it feels too late. Discussing this, she decides a next step she would like to take, regardless of the cause of her pain, is a private referral to a fertility specialist.

General conversational tool – talking with health professional patients

In our encounters with our professional colleagues, we would like to embrace their expertise and see them as a whole person. We can partner with them to discuss different ways to approach their situation and together find ways to optimise holistic health, prioritising what is important today.

Address any hierarchy, If we are acting superiorly, then we can check we have open, respectful verbal and non-verbal communication, turning our body and attention to the person and involving them, *I am interested in your thoughts about this.*

If we notice that we are acting in an inferior position, then we can adjust our posture to bring our shoulders back and use assertive language, *I need to ask a few more questions, if that's OK?*

Normalise and validate, using our shared knowledge,

> *I am glad you were able to get an appointment that worked with your schedule. It can be hard to prioritise our own health.*

Professional hat on and off. Allow the person's health professional and "off work" selves to both be present,

> *What other tests were you thinking about? When you take off your health professional hat, what goes through your mind?*

Reference

1. Balban, M.Y., Neri, E., Kogon, M.M., Weed, L., Nouriani, B., Jo, B., Holl, G., Zeitzer, J.M., Spiegel, D., & Huberman, A.D. (2023). Brief Structured Respiration Practices Enhance Mood and Reduce Physiological Arousal. Cell Rep Med. 4(1): 100895. https://doi.org/10.1016/j.xcrm.2022.100895

8

Low mood and depression

> Coming to this group helps me get out of the house and make connections. Hearing others talk has made me feel OK with sharing my story – that takes more time than primary care can give. Plus, here I get to hear what tools the others are getting from their psychologists. I am learning so much – the group is like my own therapy.
>
> **Naomi***

Introduction

Low mood and depression are common mental health problems we encounter in primary care. If we think of anxiety and depression as being at opposite ends of a continuum, most people will present along this with a mix of both.

Depression is characterised by a loss of interest and pleasure in normal experiences, low mood and a whole range of symptoms, which may be emotional, cognitive, physical and/or behavioural.

In primary care, we need to be able to recognise depression and assess its severity and impact. We need to be able to ask sensitively about self-harm and suicidal risk. Treatment may include medication, referral to psychological services, self-help and support groups, and online or written material. Follow-up and a robust safety net are important.

DOI: 10.1201/9781003409168-11

In this chapter, we consider ways to discuss and agree a plan that can start as soon as someone leaves the conversation – instead of, or while waiting for, medication to start working or an appointment with a psychologist.

We will consider three common presentations of depression in primary care and approaches to these conversations:

Example 1 – Harry Johnson, 22 years. *I feel depressed.*

Example 2 – Melissa Tomson, 27 years. Postnatal low mood.

Example 3 – Manjit Singh, 34 years. Depression.

Tools in this chapter

1   Activity layers.
2   Treasure hunt questions.
3   Significant statements.

Additional tool

•   An image or metaphor – see Chapter 5.

Activity layers

The theory that underpins activity layering is behaviour activation, an approach to mental health that uses our behaviours to influence how we feel. Most research into behavioural activation is for depression, where it has been shown to be highly effective. A systematic review found a number needed to to treat (NNT) of 2.5 for behavioural activation for depression, measured a week to a month after the interventions.[1] This suggests that behavioural activation is one of the most effective treatments for depression. A focus on "doing" adapts well to a primary care setting.

The best way to set up a new behaviour and ingrain it as a habit is by starting really small and building up, and this is a principle we apply throughout this text. The small thing we do today starts to activate neural networks, and the repetition begins to rewire our brains due to synaptic plasticity. The small action becomes easier over time until we do it automatically with minimal effort.

Treasure hunt questions

We go on a treasure hunt to find nuggets of gold – in this case, insights into how the problem is affecting the person and what is different, or missing, compared with when they felt in better health. We may use a general question to find out **how** the problem is affecting the person now, compared with "before", listening for impact. We might ask someone who has had problems for a year or so,

With all of this going on, what has life been like this last 12 months?

After hearing the answer to this general overview question, we can ask a more time-defined question, to find out the more recent impact,

What has been or felt different over the last week, compared with a similar week last year before you felt like this?

Significant statements

A significant statement may be a sweeping generalisation or a hard-hitting statement a person makes about themselves, others or the world. It may be dropped in the middle of other information, giving us an easy reason to be distracted or not notice it. Significant statements give us important information about how someone sees themselves and the world and this will influence their behaviours.

Training ourselves to notice these statements takes practice. We may well be juggling several other tasks in the conversation such as uncertain diagnoses, physical and mental health needs and safety. The first step is starting to listen out and ask ourselves, *Could that be a significant statement?*

We might use one or more tools to respond to a significant statement, such as looking for evidence for and against it being true. At other times, noticing significant statements that are getting in the way of life could lead to a discussion about the benefits of a referral for psychological therapy.

What about peer support? The quote at the beginning of this chapter refers to a peer support group. Peer support brings together a group of people who may have a shared experience of a mental health or substance use condition. People can use their own experiences to help others and provide a space where there is acceptance and understanding.

Example 1 – *I feel depressed*

In this case, we consider how to discuss and create a plan using "activity layers" for someone with low mood. When we feel low, we focus on negatives rather than positives and may be critical of ourselves and our actions. This can be a sign of a lack of self-compassion, see Chapter 13.

Tools

• Image or metaphor – phone filter.

• Activity layers.

Patient	Harry Johnson, 22 years, male.
PMH	None.
Opening statement	*Uni years are supposed to be the best years of your life but I feel depressed – the worst I ever have.*

What do you say now?

Harry has asked about a discoloured nail and now surprises us with the above statement. How should we approach this?

First, we want to understand more about Harry and this situation. Reflecting his words we ask,

Tell me a bit about feeling depressed, the worst you ever have?

Then we ask some follow-up questions,

Have others around you noticed? What would they have seen that seems different from how you usually are?

Have you had any times in the past when you have felt similar to this? What helped then? How did things get to a better place?

We find out that Harry has no friends nearby and spends a lot of free time alone. He has not yet met anyone around whom he can "be himself". His course feels overwhelming and, while he wants to pass, he has not yet started an assignment that is due soon. He is not sure what is wrong with him. In the past, he has always completed assignments on time and feels stupid to have left it so late. We reflect back what we have heard about what's important to Harry,

One thing that's making life tough, or even the worst you have known, is not having friendships. I hear this is something you really value. Things feel overwhelming and you have found it hard to take the first step to start this assignment, something I think many others have experienced at some point – I certainly have. It sounds as if there has been a lot to adjust to as normally you start assignments early. Overall, I sense you are glad to be studying this course and keen to complete it.

Harry agrees but also says his parents would "disown" him if he failed. He has this feeling because, when he speaks to them, they often ask how the course is going. He says,

I can't fail, I would be a total embarrassment to my family.

What is wrong with me, why can't I just get on with it?

In the past, he has never had these problems. Before he moved away to university, he was in a number of sports teams – these were where some of his friendships started, and he often socialised after matches. However, he doesn't want to join an established team here; he wouldn't want to force himself into somewhere he was "not welcome".

We notice some of Harry's comments seem to indicate low self-compassion. Even in this tough time with a move to a new place where he is socially isolated and on a high-pressure course, his language tells us that he has not lowered his expectations or been kind to himself. We reflect this, framing it to include specifics,

Even with the many changes you have recently navigated, with a move to a new place, new people and a new course, your expectations of yourself are to perform as you have in the past. I'm wondering if you might tend to be more critical rather than understanding of yourself?

Harry agrees and we comment,

There can be pros and cons to these high expectations – on the one hand, it could give motivation to achieve; on the other it could feel like telling our-selves we are failing. That can lead to other negative thoughts and can make it harder to start or try things. Sometimes talking to ourselves instead, like a supportive coach, can feel reassuring and make it easier to take action.

We make a note of this in our records – something to potentially come back to at a follow-up.

Safety

We decide to talk next about safety. First, we use a general open question, then a precise one,

When things have felt at their worst, what thoughts have you had?

It is very common in these situations to have thoughts like "It would be easier to fall asleep and not wake up". Have you had this type of thought? What sorts of things have you thought?

We are reassured that Harry quickly confirms that this has never been an issue and that he would talk to his parents if this did happen, as it would be really disturbing for him.

An image or metaphor

Having completed data gathering, we decide to use an image to explain some of what seems to be happening,

What can sometimes happen is that when things feel difficult – "the worst ever" – it is like having a phone camera filter applied to the world; our brain notices this and then starts to apply it more of the time. Seeing the world through a "worst" filter can be a problem because it makes us want to hide and puts us off doing or trying things.

If we realise our brain is interpreting the world with this "worst" filter on, we can perhaps step back and try to look at things without this. For example, we could try out a different filter and ask ourselves what this situation might look like with the "best" filter.

Activity layers

Inaction, as Harry has described with not starting his assignments, is very common. It can be hard to make a start. The best thing we can do is to support finding a really small first action. Indecision around if it is the "right" action may be limiting, but at this point, the emphasis is on a small step in any direction,

If we want to try a small step into life without a "worst ever" filter, to see how the world looks differently, what would be a small thing you could do?

This type of open question permits a response from any area of life, from study to social activities, wherever someone may have been contemplating a change. Harry says he was thinking of going for a jog. There is a park near him and he saw a route that others were taking – he thinks getting fitter will be good for him. Although this may well help, we might think that he would perhaps benefit even more from a sport involving others. This could be an additional activity layer that is added later.

We focus on some specifics and hold up this option to a "truth light" to see if it sounds realistic and feasible. We might use some of these,

Is that something you could do? When (day/time) would you start? How often/how long would you aim for?

Shall we decide this is what you will do and "lock it in"?

What could stop this happening? What could help get around that?

Does this feel manageable?

Harry tells us he has actually walked the route, jogging a bit here and there, and he will now do this every day. We discuss this, and it seems this would be a big increase from no regular exercise. Our goal is for the activity to be successful, and it can of course be exceeded. Harry says a walk or jog three times in the next week is realistic. He scores this as 8/10 likelihood of happening.

This was a priority area for Harry. We know this because it is one that he had both contemplated and already started taking action on. We decide to ask about a second action, related to his course,

It sounds as if a walk or jog three times in the next week on this route is something you are confident you can fit in to life. We know that exercise and being outside, in the park and around nature, are both things that contribute to a positive "filter" on the world and support our physical and mental health.

I wonder if it is the right time to also plan an action about your course and if you have any thoughts about a small first step?

Harry says he thinks he needs to contact his course tutor. Exploring this, he says he will email and try and arrange a time to meet in person as soon as possible.

Finally, if Harry is concerned about his mood or safety, or things feel worse, we ask him to contact us again or use a support phone line, including outside working hours. We make sure he has the relevant details.

Specific conversation tool – activity layers

Think of a cake that may start as a single layer, but then have a filling and additional layer(s) added. The aim of activity layers is to experiment with, and find, an activity that creates a desired impact on mood, then establish a routine including this activity. Then further activities can be added, like extra cake layers.

The activities will be either *things I need to do* or *things I want to do*. The cake filling – or way of dividing the activities – is time. In a primary care setting we may make a plan that starts with one activity a day or with completing the same activity a certain number of times in a week.

Activity ladder compared with activity layers

In our discussion of situational anxiety in Chapter 6, we described an activity ladder. There are similarities between this and activity layers; in particular, they are both behavioural or activity focused.

A difference is that in the activity ladder the second step is an expansion, **replacing** the first, bringing a person nearer to the eventual desired activity. In contrast, in activity layers the second activity is **in addition** to continuing the first, increasing the total number of activities.

Example 2 – postnatal low mood

The peri- and postnatal periods are vulnerable times for our mental health. There are many reasons for this, including physiological factors (hormone changes, sleep deprivation), birthing experiences (a birth that is different from the anticipated birth plan, the need for interventions or time on a neonatal unit, difficulties with breastfeeding and early bonding) and psychosocial factors (adjusting to a new identity and changes in relationships, social isolation, expectations of others, including contrasting cultural ideas).

Here we consider how to move from a discussion about negative thoughts and beliefs towards an action-focused next step.

Patient	Melissa Tomson, 27 years, female; with Isabella, six weeks.
PMH	Gravida 1, Para 1. Emergency lower segment caesarean section six weeks ago.
Social history	Lives with partner.
Behaviour	Looks tired and anxious.
Opening statement	*I am always tired. I can't get anything done. She is always unsettled – I can never settle her. I am not a natural mother.*

What do you say now?

We respond to this with an empathetic expression,

I'm hearing things are really tough at the moment.

Melissa spontaneously continues to talk. We listen and hear that she is frequently checking Isabella, she doesn't trust the baby monitor and her sleep has been very interrupted. She loves Isabella and feels a strong connection but worries about letting her baby down.

In this conversation, it is important to demonstrate understanding – that we have heard and understood the situation, thoughts and feelings. We use a non-judgemental, curious tone.

Without knowing any specifics, we ask,

It sounds like maybe things are different from how you expected; would that be right? In what ways?

We listen carefully. Melissa says that Isabella is always unsettled. She has now said this twice; we pick up the cue and ask,

When she is unsettled, what goes through your head?

Although Isabella seems healthy and is growing well, Melissa worries that there might be an undiagnosed problem, even though she has been reassured at the accident and emergency department (A&E). Melissa has told us twice that there is nothing she can do, *I can never settle her,* and implied that "there is a problem someone else can fix". Feeling out of control or helpless can weigh heavily and it is useful to reflect this back,

> *When you are trying everything you can to settle Isabella and nothing is working, that can feel really difficult. We can have big expectations of ourselves.*

At this point Melissa looks as if she might cry. We ask,

> *What are some of the emotions that have been coming up for you these last few weeks? It looks like there are a lot near the surface.*

Melissa feels overwhelmed and that, despite trying her best, nothing seems to be good enough. She worries about how she will cope as a mother. We acknowledge "not good enough", "worried" and "scared". We ask whether there is someone she has felt able to talk with about this. She says she has cried in the shower, but has not shared these feelings. We reflect this using normalising and positive framing,

> *You are right; it can be hard to start these conversations and reveal some of our beliefs about ourselves. It is even harder when you are tired and with everything that has been happening for you in the last few weeks. I think you have had to be strong to talk about this today.*

Metaphor – sticky negative thoughts

We now have some idea of how it feels to be in Melissa's shoes. We have developed rapport through a shared understanding of how life is day-to-day with Isabella being unsettled, and the thoughts and feelings that go with this – *I'm not good enough, not a natural mother.* We use a metaphor to further develop understanding,

> *When we start having these thoughts, "nothing I do helps", and feeling "not good enough", they can be sticky. But more positive thoughts don't stick – they are less sticky and sometimes so brief that we don't even notice them.*

Treasure hunt question

We now want to pivot to focus on positives using a treasure hunt question,

> *Tell me about a time in the last few weeks when you have felt positive?*

We develop this by asking,

What was happening then? What thoughts did you have? How did you feel? What did you do next?

Melissa thinks and tells us about holding Isabella as she slept after a feed. She was sitting comfortably and felt content and peaceful. You notice her face relaxing as she talks and reflect. You ask about where this was: is this where she usually sits, what thoughts did she have sitting there watching Isabella sleep? Melissa tells us that she felt satisfied and content that she had done a good job. She was happy sitting there in the lounge, on the sofa. Next, her partner took Isabella for a cuddle and Melissa phoned her mum whilst preparing food for dinner.

Next steps

We want to build on this positive experience and ask,

Is this something that we could plan to recreate, even though we cannot guarantee when Isabella will sleep? You mentioned that you involved your partner and your mum?

We may go on to point out that, perhaps through feeling content and that she had been a good parent, she allowed herself permission to involve others. Perhaps involving others may have a positive effect, helping create some contented feeling. We suggest that she might perhaps think positively about how many people Isabella has around her who love her and care for her.

If we felt an additional action may be useful, rather than overwhelming, we might ask about the time Melissa has for her own health and well-being,

For you to be the best parent you can be, it can be useful to have foundations in place for your health and well-being. These can help to break through the sticky thoughts, to get a better view of reality. Things like eating well, enough sleep, time outdoors, and some physical and mental stimulation. What could be a starting point for one small step with one of these?

Together, we decide a next step would be for Melissa to pursue her interest in ongoing learning. She will listen to a podcast, perhaps linked to work, whilst walking with Isabella. This would combine physical exercise, fresh air and mental stimulation.

Finally, we plan to see Melissa and Isabella in a couple of weeks to see how she is getting on. At this next consultation, she tells us she has followed through with the plan and is walking and has been listening to podcasts. She has found a postnatal depression support group and these meetings are helping her mood.

Ways to improve sleep

Any kind of stimulation activates the brain and reinforces wakefulness, making sleep less likely. External stimulation can be our baby crying, screens, food or drink. We need to avoid these when we want to be asleep.

Reduce time spent lying awake in bed – go to bed later (to reduce sleep latency) or get up if lying awake after about 20 minutes.

Check sleep hygiene – screens outside the bedroom, no clock watching, a warm shower or bath before bed, wake at a constant time every day, getting outside for 20 minutes in the morning to stimulate the serotonin-melatonin cycle through exposure to natural blue light.

For sleep, we need to feel safe and calm in mind and body. Practical steps may include a plan for delegating caring responsibilities for children or relatives, where possible, and creating a quiet, cool and dark room for sleep. Then discuss ways to create a calm body and calm mind, for example, time to write down anxieties in a "worry time" before getting into bed and breathing exercises in bed.

Remember there is no "off" button to fall asleep or a medication that can "switch our brains off". Changes take practice and time.

Example 3 – low mood

Here, we outline a way to talk about thinking. In this case, it involves negative recurring thoughts that are impacting the person's life. These may be expressed as "significant statements" that we hear in conversations. The steps we use to work with a significant statement, in this case, are:

- Identify the statement and reflect.
- Assess.
- Discuss.

Patient	Manjit Singh, 34 years, male.
PMH	Appendicectomy aged 15 years. Fractured tibia and fibula in a road accident seven years ago. Bell's palsy 11 months ago. Depression – several episodes in his 20s and recurrence 18 months ago.
Social history	Lives with wife and children, his cousin and his parents.
Medication	Sertraline 100 mg daily, started during the last episode of depression and continued.
Opening statement	*I am depressed and this medication is not working anymore.*

What do you say next?

We listen, reflect and ask open questions and find out that Manjit's mood has been low for the last few months. He has been out of work for eight months and initially thought he would find another role quickly but hasn't. This is causing financial stress at home, though with his cousin and wife's incomes, they can just about get by.

He confirms he is still exercising, which seemed to help last time when he was depressed but doesn't seem to be effective now. He is going for a short walk daily.

His sleep is fine. He enjoys time with his children. He has gained weight over the last six months, perhaps 5 kg. He feels safe and has not had thoughts of suicide. While exploring these areas, Manjit has said,

> *I have no motivation. My wife sees me going downhill and getting back to how I was before. I didn't even bother to apply for the last job I saw advertised. That is how pathetic I am. I do all the things they said last time and go through the motion of these daily walks and breathing exercises. But I can tell I am going downhill.*

Note and discuss a significant statement

We note a potentially significant statement and decide to reflect it,

> *When you were talking just now, the word "pathetic" stood out to me. Is that something that just came into your head now or something that you have thought before?*

Manjit says it is not a thought, it is a fact. No one has said it, but they don't need to. When he had time off work with depression previously, he could see it on the faces of his co-workers. He sees the same look from his cousin and parents. At meals, he is the failure in the room and knows they are thinking about how long it has been since he could contribute financially to the family.

Assess

From this we can conclude that this is a recurrent thought, and it could be affecting Manjit's life and what he is doing. To explore this significant statement's impact, we decide to zoom in to ask about what happens at mealtimes, and what impact this thought has on what he does,

When you have these thoughts about being "pathetic" or the "failure in the room", do these thoughts affect what you might normally do, for example at meals or other times?

Manjit says he avoids eye contact. He used to be the one to keep the conversation going, getting the children to talk to the other adults. These days meals are quieter. If he had a job, he would of course be himself and know his value in the house.

We ask what is important to him about mealtime conversations, and he tells of the joy it brings his parents. He grew up close to his grandparents in a multigenerational household and always valued them and his relationship with them.

Discuss

There are a number of ways we can discuss a significant statement.

Weigh up and test the statement

Would it be the case that anyone out of work for as long as you would have less value? What if it was someone who had previously been, say, the prime minister or someone else you admire? What would be different then?

Examine and explore the statement

If you were to have this thought "I am pathetic", is that something you see – as if it were written down? Or is it a voice saying it? What type of writing or voice?

What happens if we change that? If we turn down the volume so that "I am pathetic" is whispered quietly, or written in fluffy cloud writing, does anything change with how true it is or how much it affects you?

Lost in translation

We can also explore if the message is being distorted and means something else,

> *Meal times sound significant. Everyone is together, and you have an important role in helping the conversation flow. Not everyone has that skill, which is maybe why, when you don't do it, things are quieter.*

> *I wonder if, when you have this thought "I am a failure" or "I am pathetic" at mealtimes, perhaps your brain is trying to tell you something, but it's mistranslated. For example, could your brain be trying to get your attention to say, "You have an important job to do here", to help the conversation?*

"Even with"

We use another approach – "even with" – a good way to find an action to take as a next step. We ask,

> *It sounds as if your role at meals, in keeping the conversation going, is important for everyone. If we wanted to find a way for you to try doing this again, even with this thought being in your head – that "others might think I am pathetic or a failure" – what would be a small step that you could take today towards helping the mealtime conversation flow?*

Manjit mentions that he was astonished earlier this week that no one asked his son about his class assembly, and he thinks he could bring this up this evening. The principle here is that our actions affect how we feel and that changing the action – even with the thought unchanged – can affect our mood.

We summarise,

> *I know you have felt your mood is worse lately and it has been a tough time, not hearing from jobs you have applied for. In your position I would also find it hard to keep positive. You have done really well to keep up the walking every day. It could be a good time to try a small step towards restarting your mealtime role. It may feel difficult or unnatural at first and needs practice. Even though this is one small thing, sometimes changing something small like this can actually have a bigger change on how we feel.*

> *Depending on how this goes, we might think about other people who could be involved – like when you mentioned seeing a psychologist last time or medication changes – so it will be good to meet up in a week to see how things are.*

Top tips for talking about general mental health

There are things that we can do that will benefit our mental health (even if we don't feel like doing them), starting with small, realistic daily steps that we can do regularly and build into habits. For example:

- Eat a diet with a wide variety of whole foods, predominantly plant-based.
- Move our bodies regularly, in a way that works for us.
- Spend time in nature – surround ourselves with naturally occurring green and blue colours.
- Connect with others – prioritise spending time in positive relationships.
- Take time for physical and mental rest.
- Consider ways to connect with our creative, religious, spiritual and/ or cultural selves.
- Be kind to ourselves – in how we treat our bodies and what we tell ourselves, literally holding our own hand and changing self-criticism to self-compassion.

Reference

1. Ekers, D., Webster, L., Van Straten, A., Cuijpers, P., Richards, D., & Gilbody, S. (2014). Behavioural Activation for Depression: An Update of Meta-Analysis of Effectiveness and Sub Group Analysis. PLoS ONE. 9(6):e100100. https://doi.org/10.1371/journal.pone.0100100

CHAPTER

9

Young people

Introduction

> I was given medication but I didn't take it. I enjoy art. When I got referred to a cultural support group, the case worker took me to play basketball. It didn't change my situation but it was good to get out of the house, and I think it helped my mood.
>
> **Piripi★**

Young people have unique challenges affecting their emotional, physical and mental health. In adolescence, many social, physical and psychological changes occur. A sense of "self" develops, gender and sexuality are explored, and relationships with family and peers change. Potential for harm to health may come from alcohol, cannabis or other drugs, unsafe driving, social media or sexual encounters. Mental health symptoms may first manifest in young people, with higher rates in some groups such as LGBTQIA+. Loneliness may be a particular challenge that affects a young person's physical and mental health.[1]

Early experiences with health services will influence future willingness to access them. Developing effective coping strategies and positive behaviours to support mental health during adolescence can have benefits into adulthood.

Before a conversation, you may want to consider ways to make the setting feel familiar or accessible for young people. Some factors to consider may

DOI: 10.1201/9781003409168-12

include comfortable seating, access to Wi-Fi, confidentiality and privacy, access to bathrooms, use of preferred name and pronouns, and supporting a young person to have people they want present and not have those they don't want present for all or part of a conversation.

Young people have embraced virtual consulting using both phone and video for conversations. Both of these seem to be safe and helpful. These virtual conversations may provide the opportunity for a confidential discussion without parents or caregivers present.[2]

We may well, however, encourage young people to involve a parent or trusted adult and may offer to help them have these conversations. If they continue to wish to seek care alone, we need to assess their capacity to make decisions.[3]

If the young person is accompanied to a face-to-face consultation by a parent or caregiver, it is useful to have part of the conversation with everyone present and part with the young person on their own.

In the consultations that follow, we consider the conversation between the clinician and young person, without another adult being present.

Existing tools for assessing mental health in young people

There are specific tools for assessing youth well-being. These include the Patient Health Questionnaire-9 (PHQ9) for adolescents and PCAP, which is a simple model that considers protective factors for youth well-being.

PCAP model

People	Having an adult in your life who cares.
Contribution	Having opportunities to contribute to family, school/work or community.
Activities	Being involved in an activity where a sense of connection can develop.
Place	Having a safe place to be with adult supervision.

Formal or informal?

In conversations with friends and family, we may have a wide spectrum of styles – friendly, relaxed, perhaps abrupt – depending on our mood and the situation. At work, in consultations, we may adopt a "professional" mode.

Patients may already feel vulnerable before they see us – worried about their health – and our "professional" behaviour may emphasise a power imbalance. With a young person who is inexperienced at being a patient, we may want to consider ways to be more informal. For example, reducing the height of our seat, having a more open and relaxed posture or using language that we hear the young person use that may differ from our more usual professional vocabulary.

In this chapter, we use a number of tools already discussed and add some variations on these, such as a life raft and coping menu, which we may be more likely to use with young people:

Example 1 – Hugo O'Neil, 14 years. Low mood and stress.

Example 2 – Danielle Campbell, 12 years. Nausea and vomiting.

Example 3 – Josh Brown, 15 years. Grief, anger and anxiety.

Tools in this chapter

1 Coping menu.
2 Life raft.
3 What balances that?

Additional tools

- Image or metaphor – see Chapter 5
- Think, feel, do (body and you) – see Chapter 6
- Choose the focus – See Chapter 7
- Detective, judge, court reporter – see Chapter 7
- Activity layers – see Chapter 8

Coping menu

Most people will already have ways of coping with difficulties. First, we explore existing strategies,

When you start to worry about this, what do you do to cope?

We listen particularly for a range of strategies, perhaps some that involve other people and others that can be done alone, possibly including different senses such as hearing or taste. We consider whether these are transferable to other situations, particularly any specific situations mentioned. Summarising these provides a "menu" of ways to cope.

Life raft

A life raft provides refuge when at sea. We can build a life raft before we approach questions that someone may find difficult to answer or a situation where we are struggling to build rapport.

The life raft is formed from safe topics that interest a person and are easy to talk about. We find these out by experimenting – asking about friends, hobbies or future plans while closely watching for longer answers or more eye contact. Sometimes we may use a pair of questions – closed, followed by open,

Do you enjoy being part of the netball team – thumbs up or thumbs down? [closed]

Tell me about something that happened recently at netball that wasn't so great [open]

With a life raft established, we have somewhere to return to for a break if other parts of the conversation become challenging.

What balances that?

When someone expresses a strong feeling, perhaps of anger, self-blame or worthlessness, we need to find a counterbalance. We might ask, *You said that when you failed the test, you felt worthless. Balancing that, when was a time that you really felt good about yourself?* It may be helpful to find a strong and significant person to express the balancing position. This might be mum or dad, a trusted teacher or headteacher, or a youth worker. We can, metaphorically, invite this person into our conversation to provide the flipside,

What do you think X would say if they were in this room now and heard you saying that you should have done A instead of B?

In our experience, even if they feel strong emotions, people can give themselves positive reinforcement when asked to see the situation through the eyes of a trusted and valued person.

Example 1 – low mood and stress

Patient	Hugo O'Neill, 14 years.
PMH	Rarely attends. Recent letters from a transgender clinic. Skateboarding injury last week – checked at A&E, nil serious.
Social history	Lives with both parents and younger brother.
Behaviour	Quiet, seems reluctant to talk. Looks down.
Opening statement	*The school nurse said I should get this cut checked out.*

What do you say next?

Getting a conversation off to a good start with a young person can include taking time to learn something about their identity by checking their preferred name and pronouns. We decide to model this for them,

Hi, I am Sophie. I am a nurse working here. I use the pronouns she/her. I prefer if you call me Sophie but "nurse", "Sophie" or "nurse Sophie" are all fine. How about you? What name do you prefer? How about pronouns?

Hugo tells us he prefers to be called Myth and uses the pronouns "they/them". The wound does not seem infected and is healing well. There are no other injuries. We notice Myth speaks quietly with short answers and decide to ask about mental health. Myth seems reluctant to talk and, because of this, we use a life raft.

We know Myth is attending school and spends time skateboarding. These are potentially safe topics and could be a conversational life raft. We start with factual questions and also remember that questions about other people, such as friends or family, may be easier. By doing this, we hope Myth will gain confidence so that we can move into other topics,

When did you start skateboarding? How often do you do this?

How did you first get into it? What do your friends think about it?

We notice that we are establishing a life raft because Myth relaxes a little and increases their eye contact.

Moving on and off a life raft

With a life raft established we move on to another topic and used paired closed and open questions,

How's school? What's good and what's not so good? Can you tell me about something recently that was not so good?

We listen closely, paying attention to body language and allowing pauses to allow Myth time to respond if they want,

The nurse at school asked if I do drugs.

We have noted distress in Myth's voice, so, rather than leaping into this difficult subject, we respond with a statement and then use the life raft, offering a question with two potential responses,

Some people try drugs as an experiment or in response to feelings like being anxious or depressed.

Hey, with your skateboarding, are you working on a particular skill, or do you prefer to just do what you feel on the day, or something else?

Myth tells us that they like skateboarding. They are good with the basics and like board designs. We now return to the more difficult topic, starting with a reflection on the easier topic. Then we socially distance the difficult question, e.g. "people at your school". We may follow up by bringing this nearer, "any of your friends?",

You want to keep skateboarding enjoyable, not too intense.

You know how the nurse asked you about drugs? Do you think many people at your school do drugs?

Myth tells us that some people at school smoke, including their friends, but they are not interested in trying drugs and are upset that adults keep asking. Does everyone think the worst of them? We respond,

It's annoying to have to repeat yourself. It is possible that people around you want to keep you safe and maybe want to let you know that you can talk to them about stuff like drugs or your mood.

Who would you say are the people you can turn to if you need support?

Myth identifies friends from their previous school as their main support and, if an adult had to be involved, their older sister, Kate, who has left home. They changed schools at the start of this year because of moving house. They tell us that they are closer to their previous school friends because they used to do stuff together, but they can't really be bothered to contact them now.

Myth has got into a habit of going home from school and spending the rest of the day alone in their bedroom. They stay on their device late into the night and then struggle to get to sleep.

Image or metaphor – brain texting error messages

This may be a useful metaphor for young people, because many, from increasingly young ages, have mobile phones. Most of us have experienced an error when texting. Perhaps we sent a message to the wrong person or sent a message with a single typo that completely alters the meaning (e.g. "not" for "now"). When we are busy or stressed due to the volume of communication, errors can be more likely.

In the same way, we have constant communication with our brains. Our brain tells us when we feel hungry or tired. But does it always send the correct message?

> *I really can't be bothered to go for a run tonight, I'm just too tired.*

However, we go for a run and afterwards feel more energetic. This initial message was like a texting error. There was never supposed to be a "t" after the "can".

We decide to use this metaphor, as Myth has told us that they "can't be bothered" or "don't feel like" doing things after school. We would intersperse this information with conversation and check understanding,

> *You know something I find interesting: our brains send us messages all day long, for example "Don't cross the road until after that car". Sometimes they send a message that is an error – like sometimes we hit the wrong key and send someone a different emoji than the one we intended or send the right message but to the wrong person. Have you ever done that? I have.*

> *A message like "I can't be bothered to contact my friends" could be a real message. Maybe you had a really busy day and could do with a rest, but it could also be an error. This can feel like a strange idea – our brains getting things wrong – but it happens to us all. Maybe you have felt hungry but then become busy and realise later you were bored, not hungry.*

Turning the metaphor into an action plan

As Myth seems engaged and thoughtful about this, we decide to continue and move to a plan. With metaphors or images, we are mindful that if someone does not seem to relate to them, we will put them aside. We might then simply mention that the thought "I can't be bothered" could be true or not true, and we wouldn't know until we try.

Here, we continue with the metaphor and say,

> *How can we know if it is an error message or if we should listen to our brain and "not bother"? The only way to be sure is to get to understand more about how your brain works. This means trying out the activity even when you have noted a "can't be bothered" message and noticing how you feel before, during and after.*

> *If you contact your friends and, after a chat on the phone, notice you feel a little more energy or more content in yourself, then you might conclude the "can't be bothered" message was an error. Knowing this can be useful for next time.*

If we think Myth would like some science behind this, we might explain that we can "rewire" our brains over time by continuing the activity despite the message. Although it may still be present for a while, the message gradually lessens because of neuroplasticity. This idea – of rewiring and structural changes in response to what we do – may be novel to Myth and may help understanding and motivation.

Activity layers

So far, we have learnt about positive activities and people, connections with friends from a previous school, their sister, skateboarding and time in Myth's own safe space (bedroom).

We decide to build an activity layers plan based on the following questions:

- What can I do?
- Who can support me?
- What's my backup?

What can I do?

> *Are there other things you can do when you can't skateboard or if your old friends don't answer a text or call?*

We may prompt,

> *Being physically active outside is really good for our health. Is there any other activity you could do, if for some reason you had to stay inside?*

Myth says they like to design patterns to decorate skateboards. They haven't for a while but have the materials they need. They think this would be achievable – to get the drawing pad out, look through previous designs and select those that most appeal to them today.

Who can support me?

Myth would like to contact Zack from primary school, but he is not always quick at replying. Myth will try again and be patient, accepting that the reply might be slow, rather than assuming that Zack doesn't want to return the contact.

What's my backup?

Myth could phone their sister, Kate, as she would call back and not pressurise them to talk about anything they didn't want to and has called them back before, even late at night. Together you work out the words for a text for Myth to send to Kate.

We now have some layers of an activity layer cake:

- **Doing active** – skateboarding.
- **Doing quiet** – colouring.
- **Contacting** – primary school friend.
- **Backup** – sister.

We have discussed trying these activities, even when messages like *I can't be bothered* come from their brain, as a way of enabling Myth to understand themself better and what kind of error messages their brain might send and at what times.

We might summarise this plan,

> *It is great you have skateboarding that you enjoy and have time to do this, particularly at weekends. It would be good to see if re-starting the colouring and meeting up with a couple of your primary school friends make any change to your mood. Can we plan to speak again? For now, you have your sister as a backup and, if needed, this number is a 24/7 helpline.*

Learning point – avoidance

We can probably all relate to the "solution" of avoidance. *If I don't do it, I won't feel anxious*, or *If I am not in class, I can't vomit in front of my peers*, or as Myth has told us, *I can't be bothered*, and they stay alone in their bedroom after school.

(Continued)

Staying in bed, pulling the duvet up and hiding away from the world can be tempting – particularly if life is stressful or busy and even more so with anxiety or low mood. However, avoidance provides only a short-term fix. Coping by avoidance may maintain and even increase anxiety. We can feel worse for avoiding the problem; we may also feel guilty and the avoidance may create conflict in relationships.

Listen out in conversations for people who have had time away from work or avoided a situation. Anticipate that returning may be difficult and discuss a plan. Exposure is a core element of CBT. Taking even a small active step can reduce how big the problem feels, which can reduce anxiety and improve mood.

If there is a particular situation or activity that is being avoided, then consider using an activity ladder. This provides a way to start graded exposure from a small first step up to complete the desired activity.

Example 2 – nausea and vomiting

In this case, we consider coping strategies for physical symptoms. We also recognise the potential role of the gut microbiome and effect of the neuro-endocrine system on mood and gastrointestinal system.

Tools

- Detective, judge and court reporter.
- Coping menu.

Patient	Danielle Campbell, 12 years, female – she/her.
PMH	Intermittent nausea and vomiting for two years. Letter from paediatrics – all investigations normal. Reassured.
Social history	Lives with mum.
Opening statement	*I keep feeling sick.*

What do you say now?

Background

Danielle has had six weeks of intermittent diffuse abdominal discomfort and nausea that does not stop her from doing anything. It is more a churning sensation than pain. She had the same problem a year ago and was

143

assessed by the paediatricians. We examine her tummy and everything feels normal. We note the letter from paediatrics with negative investigations and decide to discuss mental health.

Detective, judge and court reporter (Identify, assign, discuss)

How can we start this conversation? We decide to use a tool to introduce any worries or anxiety alongside the physical symptoms – the detective, judge and court reporter. As a reminder:

- Detective – finds out facts.
- Judge – assigns responsibility.
- Court reporter – summarises and shares.

The detective

Being the detective, we want to introduce a second conversation around worries about the physical symptoms.

We use ICE questions to find out about her thoughts and worries,

> *What thoughts have you had about the pain and nausea? What do you think might happen with these in the future? What worries you most about having nausea and pains?*

Danielle tells us she is worried about vomiting in front of her class. She sits near the classroom door in case she needs to run to the bathroom and always has her eyes on the teacher so she can ask. She has never actually vomited at school. She keeps nausea medication in her pocket and often feels to check they are there. She has taken this medication at school twice in the last month. She would rather not go to school at all and avoid the chance of vomiting in class but is "forced to go".

The detective has now found out the facts – never vomited at school, nausea, needing medication twice in the last month, sitting near the door, alert for teacher and medication checking, stopping concentration on work, worries about vomiting in front of class.

The judge

With this information, we can weigh the effects of the physical symptoms and the worries to help focus our management plan:

- Physical symptoms – nausea, medication needed twice.
- Worries – sitting near the door, looking out for the teacher, not concentrating, checking pocket.

The court reporter

Now, as the "court reporter", we summarise and say,

The nausea has got in the way at school at times and meant you have needed medication.

Worries about what might happen, like vomiting, are having a big impact, meaning you check the medication and stay aware of where your teacher is.

Coping menu

We move to consider coping tools, starting by exploring existing strategies,

When you start to worry about vomiting, what do you do?

Danielle tells us that she feels in her pocket to check that she has the medication by touching the packet. She also looks around for where the teacher is in the classroom – kinaesthetic and visual strategies.

We build on these existing strategies by discussing things she might notice when she looks around, as well as the teacher. We could suggest noticing the number of things that are a certain shape or counting the number of things that are shades of a particular colour.

Danielle tells us she sometimes distracts herself by pulling a hairband around her wrist, another kinaesthetic strategy. We therefore move away from visual ideas and instead ask,

Something to touch helps you cope with the feelings of nausea and tummy pain. Would there be other things you could physically touch or feel that might help?

Danielle volunteers that she has never been bothered by symptoms when relaxing and watching the TV at home. She usually lies on the sofa, cuddling her cat with a soft blanket. She thinks she could also try stretching.

The aim of these strategies is to move the focus away from the physical body sensations of anxiety, which for Danielle are nausea and tummy pain, driven by the sympathetic nervous system. Instead, the focus moves to other visual, touch or sound stimuli external to her body, which are more likely to activate the parasympathetic system. A summary of the menu of coping tools we discuss with Danielle could include:

- Severe nausea – medication and breathing.
- Worries about vomiting – physically stretching, pulling her hairband.
- Mild worries about vomiting – thinking about her cat, having something soft with her to hold.

Information giving – physiological explanation – stress mode vs relaxation mode

Some young people will be interested in an explanation of how we understand mental and physical health symptoms. This is a way to bring together the two conversations above in a way that reflects the real, complex interactions between physical and mental health.

We may explain that our brain looks out for threats or danger. If it thinks it has found a threat, it responds by producing hormones to enable our body to go into stress mode,

> Our brain and gut communicate closely using chemical messengers and are even directly connected to each other by a specific nerve. Nausea can be a response to stress as the body redirects blood from the gut to the muscles, in case we need to run away.

We might explain that the counterbalance to "stress mode" is our relaxation mode or the parasympathetic system. We explain to Danielle that this might be why she feels relaxed when lying on the sofa cuddling her cat, as this will send calm signals to her brain. We have heard that she does not feel nauseous in this calmer state. This might help us make a link – that at least part of the nausea might be related to her body going into "stress mode".

Specific conversational tool – what balances that?

This tool identifies a distressing thought, feeling or memory and seeks to balance it with another thought that creates calm feelings,

> When you notice yourself getting caught up in this (feeling/ thought/memory/worry), what could you think instead to balance this view?

(Continued)

What thought would be the opposite of this thought?

You think you have not done enough, but what's the other side of the coin, a different view, to balance this?

What would your relative/friend say about this? Does this balance the other thought?

Reframe

If you wanted to tell yourself this same thought in a different way/from a different angle, what would that be? Sometimes we might need to reframe from what we have heard,

You are spending a lot of time thinking you should have done more. You feel guilty and angry. I wonder if another way of looking at this would be to think about how you did do everything you could and would have done more if you had a chance or been asked. Could you sometimes balance your thoughts with, "I did everything I could in the situation"?

Finding the balance through values

You often think that you are a bad parent. Could it be that your brain is trying to remind you that being as good a parent as you can is important to you, and this is the more significant message?

Now you have a choice. When you notice this thought, you might decide to balance it by spending time thinking about the other view.

We use this approach in the next example.

Example 3 – grief, anger and avoidance

Here, we discuss approaches to grief. Sadness and loss can predominate and there may be anger and sometimes self-blame. We consider a way to explore these emotions and how to make a plan, working with these feelings and the difficulties they may bring.

Tools

- What balances that?

Additional tools

- Choose the focus.
- Image or metaphor.
- Think, feel, do (body and you).

Patient	Josh Brown, 15 years, male – he/him.
	Auntie is in the waiting room.
PMH	Recent hospital cardiology clinic visit.
	Attended for electrocardiogram (ECG) but
	left. Letter asks GP to rearrange.
Social/family history	Mother died 12 months ago – sudden cardiac
	event. Lives with dad. Auntie lives nearby.
Behaviour	Quiet and downcast.
Opening statement	*I just couldn't go through with it* (having the ECG).

What do you say next?

How do we approach this? Firstly, we need to rule out, as far as possible, any significant or urgent cardiac issue.

Having discovered that Josh feels well and has no physical symptoms, we move to explore what happened at the hospital using think, feel, do. We may ask one or some of these,

> Think – *When you saw the machine and wanted to leave, what thoughts were going through your head?*
>
> Feel – *Did you notice any particularly strong emotions while you were at the hospital?*
>
> Do – *What did you notice in your body? When you had this thought that you wanted to leave, what was the first thing you did?*

Josh tells us he was nervous about going to the hospital then, when he saw the machine and was asked to get on the bed, he felt overwhelmed. He wanted to get out of there. We ask, using a statement as a question so that it is easier to answer (or not, as he chooses),

> *I wonder if there have been other situations when you might have felt similar to this.*

We learn that he had been at the hospital when his mum died and had seen her with the same machine nearby. As he talks his voice becomes slightly louder and deeper. We wonder if this change is a sign of feeling anger and ask,

> *It must have brought up a lot of emotions seeing your mum like that. What feeling do you notice when we are talking now?*
>
> *I wonder if there is some anger in there, too. That would be very normal for anyone in your situation.*

Josh tells us he feels sad but then, with the prompting comment above, he agrees that sometimes he feels angry, too. We notice his jaw clenching,

> *What other thoughts go through your head when you feel angry about all this?*

Josh tells us he overheard some relatives talking and it sounded like maybe there had been a delay at the hospital. Perhaps someone else was treated first, and one of the doctors was delayed in arriving. Maybe things could have been different.

We ask who he feels most angry with. Josh says he had a headache that day but had a test, so he went to school anyway. If he had stayed at home – like his mum had asked if he needed to – they would have been together, and he could have made sure she got seen in time. We reflect that Josh's mum is very important to him and they have a special, deep connection.

What balances that?

We need a person with influence to counter a strong view of anger or self-blame. At this point we might use the idea of mum entering this conversation in order to discover the thought that would be the "flip side" of this one. We ask,

> *What do you think mum would be saying if she was in this room now and heard you saying that you should have stayed home instead of going to school?*

When asked to see things through the eyes of a valued person, it can be easier to see a positive side to a decision or action. This can be helpful to reflect,

> *When your brain is blaming you and making you feel guilty, are these words from mum – that she was glad you went to school and did the test,*

and got a good grade, because you are everything to her and she wants you to do well as school and be the best you can be – something to remember to think about?

Choose the focus

Having gained an understanding of the emotions Josh is experiencing, we next explore their impact and some options for coping,

We have talked about different feelings coming up when you think of mum. Feeling sad, lonely and angry at yourself and others. Do you think there is one of these that is happening most often or bothering you most?

Josh says that he sees things that remind him of his mum when he is in his room. He finds himself lost in memories, which are happy, but then feels sad and may cry. We ask what he does when he feels like this. He tells us he sometimes walks over to his auntie's or sits with his dad in the living room. When he feels angry, particularly with himself, he paces around his bedroom and punches his pillow. Once, he shouted at another boy at school; normally he wouldn't have reacted, but he couldn't stop himself. We reflect,

Anger can be a high-energy emotion and may come on suddenly and unexpectedly so that we can feel out of control. You may need to let it out by moving around in some way. Deciding to move can be useful, as it can remind us that we are in control of our body and what we are doing.

Sometimes anger can really take over and almost sweep you away, blaming yourself and others and wishing you could go back in time. It can be helpful if, when you notice all those thoughts and feelings, you come out of your head and remind yourself where you are physically. Notice where you are, pay attention to the physical place where you are. What can you see and hear around you?

Image or metaphor – choose the focus

We could liken this focus on feeling angry to the portrait setting on a phone camera – everything else is blurred or unseen. We want to refocus on a wider view, with many things in focus. This way we can still see and feel the anger and negative thoughts but can also see the bigger picture: other people, other feelings and other thoughts.

We use this phone metaphor with Josh,

Have you ever used the portrait setting for taking a photo on your phone? This focus on feeling angry and thinking about what could have been different is like your brain going into "portrait mode". Everything else is blurred.

What we want to do is refocus on the wider picture, even a panoramic view, where our brain can still experience this anger and blame, but can also focus on other people, many more details about what happened and what is happening around us in that moment.

These strategies are based on ACT (mindfulness) of being in the present moment and noticing the place, sounds, sights and sensations. This is a way to grow our attention to include these as well as the anger. Thus, we proportionately shrink the anger and promote the thought that we are in control and can get through, which can allow feelings of calm.

Past or present tense?

Here, although Josh's mum is no longer living, we refer to her and her voice in the present tense. This will help Josh to retain vital memories and give permission to have ongoing conversations with her.

Information giving – explaining physiology

In a follow-up conversation, we may explain that it is normal when our brain detects danger for it to want us to leave at once,

It was normal for your brain to link the machine with danger because of the experience of seeing mum linked to a machine. Anger often comes up when there is danger because of the "fight–flight" response that our body uses to keep us safe. Your brain thinks there is danger, but this machine can give us information that might help keep you safe and healthy.

Activity ladder option

We have prioritised addressing Josh's mental health and grieving. We could use an activity ladder to plan with Josh a way to build up to have this test. We could combine each step, such as looking at the room where the ECG might happen, with thinking about a time when he has felt calm or something he could do to feel more relaxed, like walking around the room rather than standing in one place.

Summary

We summarise the plan. Josh decides that when he is in his room and gets distressed by being very sad and angry, he will try counting how many different shades of blue he can see – blue was his mum's favourite colour. He thinks he could come and see the nurse in the practice to find out about what having an ECG involves. We plan a review appointment about a week after this. We finish by checking a safety plan, confirming that Josh has never had thoughts of self-harm or suicide and that he has a 24/7 contact number for support, if ever needed.

Top tips for talking with young people about mental health

Our tone and the language we use can help build rapport and help a young person feel at ease. We may use their language of nouns and verbs, if necessary, checking with the young person that we have the meaning or context correct.

In our teenage years we develop our identity and sense of self and are thinking about our future. Relationships outside the family and independence will be important. We can show our understanding and respect by asking identity questions such as: Is *there an ethnicity or culture you identify with? Would you say you have a spiritual or religious side? Have you thought about your gender/sexual identity? What thoughts have you had?*

We use "life rafts" with young people. These are topics the young person is more easily able to talk about. We would always find a life raft before starting or continuing a potentially challenging conversation so we have somewhere safe to return to, if needed.

References

1. Surkalim, D.L., Luo, M., Eres, R., Gebel, K., van Buskirk, J., Bauman, A., et al. (2022). The Prevalence of Loneliness across 113 Countries: Systematic Review and Meta-analysis. BMJ. 376:e067068. https://doi.org/10.1136/bmj-2021-067068
2. Proulx-Cabana, S., Segal, T.Y, Gregorowski, A., Hargreaves, D., & Flannery, H. (2021). Virtual Consultations: Young People and Their Parents' Experience. Adolesc Health Med Ther. 12:37–43. https://doi.org/10.2147/AHMT.S292977
3. https://www.gmc-uk.org/ethical-guidance/ethical-guidance-for-doctors/0-18-years/making-decisions/ [accessed 15 September 2023]

10

Older adults

I know him dying was my fault. I should have done something more. I have seen loads of counsellors. Thinking, *I did everything I could have in the situation I was in* – I had never looked at it like that before. On that day that thought gave me peace.

Junior*

Introduction

Older adults experience the same mental health problems that affect people of all ages. These may be compounded by issues related to ageing, such as declining physical health, loneliness and bereavement, anxiety about the future and dying, sleep problems and financial worries. "Loss" may be a prominent feature – of health, independence, one's life partner, connections with work and family, and control.

Older people may have chronic illnesses that need monitoring, or they may simply appreciate contact with a friendly and welcoming service. As with all patients we see regularly, there can be the risk of failing to notice a gradual decline in functioning or an insidious depression or assuming that symptoms are due to a known health problem rather than a new one.

Overlapping physical and mental health symptoms may present at any age, including the older populations. For example:

- **Physical symptoms caused by mental health issues**, e.g. tingling fingers caused by hyperventilation due to anxiety.

- **Physical symptoms with a physical health cause**, e.g. tingling toes caused by diabetic or alcohol-induced peripheral neuropathy.
- **Mental health issues such as health anxiety** meaning a heightened awareness of normal bodily functions that are interpreted as symptoms, e.g. a normal occasional awareness of heartbeat interpreted as palpitations.
- **Mental health issues that have caused physical health problems**, e.g. severe anxiety self-managed with heavy nicotine smoking that has caused ischaemia.
- **Conditions with significant intertwined mental, physical, cultural or social interactions**, such as irritable bowel connected with low mood due to elder abuse.

In this chapter, we will consider three common presentations:

Example 1 – Ken Davies, 76 years. Low mood and anxiety.

Example 2 – Betty Waldegrave, 83 years, and her son, Phil. Terminal diagnosis and hopelessness.

Example 3 – Anil Shah, 66 years. Grief and low mood.

Tools in this chapter

1 Problem-solving.
2 Shrink it.

Additional tools

- Image or metaphor – see Chapter 5.
- Coping questions – see Chapter 6.
- Detective, judge, court reporter – see Chapter 7.
- Choose the focus – see Chapter 7.
- Activity layers – see Chapter 8.
- Treasure hunt questions – see Chapter 8.
- What balances that? – see Chapter 9.
- Life raft – see Chapter 9.

Problem-solving

Problem-solving seeks to address issues related to life stress and find solutions to concrete issues. It is something many of us do without realising, for example,

You still need to be able to get to the shops even with your restricted mobility issues. Let's sort out access to disabled parking.

At other times we may follow a more formal process of helping someone consider their current and longer-term priorities.

Shrink it

The tool or slogan "shrink it" can be applied in any situation where either we or the person we are talking to seem to be feeling overwhelmed, uncertain or unsafe. Shrink it can mean shrinking the volume of issues or the time period being considered, or reducing the time until follow-up. It may mean we focus on the biggest problems that have come up today and ways to address these in the next 24 hours.

A variation of "shrink it", particularly where there are safety concerns, is "shrink the time, grow the team".

Example 1 – low mood and anxiety

In this example, we first want to understand more about the impacts of physical compared with mental health symptoms. We use activity layers to plan the next steps.

Tools

- Detective, judge and court reporter.
- Treasure hunt questions.
- Activity layers.

Patient	Ken Davies, 76 years, male.
PMH	Osteoarthritis (OA) spine, chronic pain. Hip replacement three months ago. Readmission two months ago with urinary sepsis. Pulmonary embolism.
Social history	Widowed four years ago. Lives alone.
Behaviour	Scruffily dressed, unshaven. Mood flat.
Opening statement	*Everything is difficult, I can't hang the washing out without stopping every few minutes – soon I won't even be able to wipe my bum.*

What do you say now?

First impressions

We immediately notice Ken's appearance, which is different from a few months ago. After exploring the pain and excluding red flags, we sense how different life is now compared with the past. We use "detective, judge, court reporter" to consider the roles of his physical and mental health, in this case his back and hip pains and mobility issues, as well as anxiety and lack of motivation.

Treasure hunt questions

We initially use treasure hunt questions,

What are some things that are different in your life now compared with before the hip problems and time in hospital?

What are you still doing that you were doing before?

Detective, judge and court reporter

The **detective's** role is to find out what is different. We find that Ken's mobility is worse, and he may need a hip replacement on the other side. Things around the house are taking longer. He worries about falling and ending up in hospital. He has not been out to his usual clubs – choir and bowls.

The **judge** asks clarifying questions in order to attribute blame or responsibility. We work out that his mobility is similar to or perhaps better than before the surgery and the pain has improved; however, he worries about falling and being readmitted to hospital. He is moving cautiously and things are taking longer.

The **court reporter** shares this information,

It sounds like day-to-day life is different from before the time in hospital. Your mobility is similar, and overall the pain is better, but your confidence has been shaken. Some things are taking longer while you get used to doing them again, but you have stuck with it – for example getting through the washing.

Coping – life experience

Someone of Ken's age has a lifetime of experience in tackling problems. We might explore previous coping strategies,

In the past, have there been times when you were trying to get through something difficult?

In that difficult time when your wife died, what were the things that helped you cope?

Ken tells us that regularly playing bowls on a Wednesday with old friends helped.

Activity layers

Now we can start to layer activities. The goal is to have a plan for specific activities on different days and times in the week. They need to be achievable, which may mean breaking them down into manageable chunks. The focus is on "doing",

Thinking about some of the things that you have enjoyed or that have helped you cope in the past, or perhaps something new, what might you think about starting or restarting?

Next, we break it down,

Taking it at a pace that works for now, what small step might be possible, leading towards these? Something that might be important to you to get done?

Self-care may be a good place to start. Daily activities that he may have previously taken for granted, such as getting up, dressing, washing and meals, are now a struggle.

We can break these down – for example prioritising getting up and eating breakfast, with dressing happening later in the day.

Ken has told us it is important to him that he is independent, but he has stopped changing his bed and washing his bedsheets. We discuss a way to resume his washing, initially in stages.

Mental exertion, physical exercise and social contact

We may consider other areas, such as mental exertion, physical exercise and social contact. He tells us he enjoys a weekly crossword. Then we ask,

Who do you like being with? If you were going to get in touch with someone, who might that be? Someone from bowls or a relative or perhaps someone you used to see?

Together we agree an achievable plan that considers both Ken's needs and the things he wants to do. "Wants" can be placed after "needs" as an incentive or reward.

Monday – AM	Take off bed sheets. Do Sunday crossword.
Monday – PM	New bed sheets on. Have afternoon tea in front of the TV.
Wednesday – PM	Phone John from bowls to ask about how the morning session went.
Thursday – AM	Wash bed sheets. Hang out washing on line (or use tumble drier).
Saturday – AM	Phone daughter.
Sunday – AM	Phone great niece.

There are spaces in the week because we want to set Ken up for success with a focus on what's important to him – getting his bed sheets changed – and looking at small steps to achieve this. Over time, additional layers will help improve Ken's physical and mental health. It is important to be realistic; even the simple plan above may need to be broken down further to ensure it is manageable. We would consider other social services that could support Ken and his goal of maintaining independence.

Some people will be able to layer activities themselves and continue with this approach. When someone has lost confidence as in this case, then we may look for other team members in health or social care who can regularly check in, support and encourage Ken.

Life events

Life events are associated with mood disorders. A particularly stressful life event may be linked with a first episode of depression. It is useful to listen for, or ask about, life events as potential triggers for physical and mental ill health. When interpreting life events, we should consider social and cultural contexts.

Some life events that can cause particular stress are the death of a loved one, job loss, moving house, divorce, major illness or injury. Other events, such as having children or retirement, are also significant and can cause anxiety or low mood.

Stressful events impact physical and mental health, illustrated by a study showing an increase in cardiovascular events after the World Trade Centre attack in 2001.[1] Identifying a recent life event should be a prompt for us to review both mental and physical health.

Example 2 – terminal diagnosis and hopelessness

In primary care, we may encounter intertwined physical and mental health issues and may need to integrate the management of several problems simultaneously. Here, with limited mobility and physical health, we focus on using creativity and imagination, introducing two tools that use visualisation.

Tools

- Safety – shrink it.
- What balances that?
- Choose the focus.
- Image or metaphor.

Patient	Betty Waldegrave, 83 years, female. Accompanied by her son, Phil.
PMH	Long-standing depression for >30 years, on a variety of medications.
	Terminal diagnosis – lung cancer with metastases – diagnosed eight weeks ago. Back pain.
Medication	Paracetamol.
Social history	Widowed many years ago. Lives in a care home. Smoker, 20 per day.
Behaviour	Sad. Exudes an air of despair.
Opening statement from her son Phil	*No one is helping her, something needs to be done, she can't go on.*

What do you say next?

There is a lot going on right from the start of this conversation including Betty's physical and mental health needs and the dynamic of their relationship. Phil might be feeling overwhelmed with emotions – helpless, distressed by his mother's pain and prognosis, anxious about how to cope with the situation. He may already be grieving the loss he will soon experience – and all this on top of anything else going on in his life. We don't know at this point how Betty is feeling or her priorities, which may be similar to or different from Phil's. With potential safety issues, we want to "grow the team", so having someone else present is helpful.

Managing more people in a safety conversation

Firstly, how do we determine who knows what and how do we navigate this? We may want to formally decide who is going to be present for different parts of this conversation. We need to consider family dynamics and culture. We may start to try and understand this by saying,

> We have lots to discuss. We can all talk together, and we may also decide to have some time where I can talk with each of you separately. How much do you talk to each other about your health/life overall?

> What about things that are difficult to discuss? In the past, have you talked to each other about anything like that?

All these questions enable dialogue between the two people, so that we can observe power dynamics and whether there seems willing agreement. If we are unsure about the interactions, we may ask to start without the relative and use this time to establish what is OK to share and discuss together. We can offer to advocate for the person and share their views if they have felt unable to do this with their relative.

If we decide to continue with both people present, we may gently move in to ask about safety,

> Have either of you been worried about Betty's safety this week?

> When things are feeling a struggle, we know people may find they have thoughts about dying. Is that something you have talked about together?

Betty says that she would like to talk to us without Phil. During this conversation, now that Phil has left the room, we notice that we start to feel overwhelmed, and we decide to use "shrink it" to ask more about safety,

> Has there been a time recently, maybe even today or yesterday, when you thought of ending your life?

Betty tells us this thought is often in her head and has been for many years. She does not feel she would act on this, but she feels hopeless because there is no future other than worsening symptoms of the cancer. We follow up by using shrink it again and asking about more positive times,

> In the last few days, when has there been a time when you have not had this thought? Perhaps when you felt a little more content.

Betty struggles to tell us anything she enjoys day-to-day; she might watch TV or listen to the radio, and the thoughts of a bleak future or suicide would usually lessen if she becomes engaged in a show.

We could follow up with a treasure hunt question and ask what was different in the past. She tells us that she used to do puzzles, but her eyesight is no longer good enough. She was also more in touch with her family, but now her daughter has moved away and her grandchildren are older and busy with their own lives.

What balances that?

We decide to prioritise a discussion about her mental health, finding a focus beyond the emotions of despair and hopelessness. First, we summarise what Betty has told us, then we use the "What balances that?" tool,

Some of the things you have enjoyed in the past have become more difficult, or not possible, as your health has changed. It seems that when nothing much is happening, for example the radio is on but you are not very interested in the topic, your brain thinks about your life ending.

Let's put these fears for the future and wanting to die on one side of a coin. Now if we imagine that we want to flip this coin over and find a memory or feeling that contrasts these, what could that be?

Betty tells us she used to think about her late sisters and some of the times as teenagers in the 1950s when they would get ready together to go out to a dance. She hasn't thought about this in a while. We ask some more questions about the dances, aiming to grow these memories and make them brighter and bigger. Does she remember music or hairstyles? She tells us she has some photos somewhere.

Image or metaphor – choose the focus

If we notice Betty changing her tone or body language, even slightly, we may comment on this,

Your brain has a lot of time to think. These thoughts about the end of your life are really dominating. Mostly you feel a sense of hopelessness or despair, feeling trapped with no way out.

In contrast to this, when thinking about times with your sisters when you were young, you mentioned feeling sad, but I noticed when you talked about that your voice changed, and I wonder if there is some happiness or fondness there, too?

Finally, we might explain,

> *Sometimes we might choose to give our brain a change from all of this think-ing and feeling of despair. A balance could be spending some time thinking about something different, like these memories of getting ready for the dance.*
>
> *Even if part of your brain tells you things like, "What's the point in think-ing about this? It won't turn back time", it can be useful to allow those thoughts and the feelings to have a place and be there like a photo or picture on the counter. You can choose to bring another photo to the front and give more attention to that one for a while.*
>
> *Perhaps you could even think about sharing these memories with Phil or maybe your grandchildren. If they are teenagers now, they might be inter-ested to learn something they never knew about you or your sisters when you were a similar age.*

Our aim here is to give a little hope that, day-to-day, perhaps things could be different and there could be a way to have a break from the persistent thoughts about dying. Perhaps this change may provide a new dimension for Phil or other relatives' relationships with Betty.

The aim is not to "delete" or "avoid" the bothersome thoughts. We acknowledge that they are still there. However, there may be a new flexibility around how intrusive they are.

Finally, after discussing it with Betty, we decide to conclude the conversa-tion with Phil present. We review their current safety plan of Phil regularly contacting Betty and suggest that we meet Betty again in the next few days to review her and see how she finds this "thought balancing".

Although Betty frequently has thoughts of hopelessness, she does not have a specific plan to end her life and also has an appointment with the hospice team, including a counsellor, the following day.

Specific conversational tool – choose the focus

When you notice that you are getting caught up in this (feeling/thought/ memory/worry), what do you do? Does it help? Have you tried anything else?

(Continued)

Connect with self

Purposeful movement – *have you tried moving in some way, for example getting up or opening and closing your hand into a fist, as a reminder that you are actually in control even though it feels that this thought is taking over?*

Have you tried using your senses to notice other different thoughts/ feelings? Using our senses of smell, sound and taste can communicate directly to our brain. Singing, humming or even gargling may all help.

Connect with values

When you notice getting caught up in this, is there a way you could remind yourself of the things most important to you?

Connect with place

Have you tried noticing where you are, for example counting shades of a particular colour that you can see? Or noticing any three things you can see, hear and feel, then two different things you can see, hear and feel and then one of each.

These can remind us that while there is a lot going on inside us – with a certain thought or memory – there are also things going on outside of us.

Imagination

When you notice being very caught up in this thought/feeling/memory/ worry, imagination can help. Perhaps imagine you are packaging up these thoughts and putting them away somewhere in a box or at the back of a drawer. Or changing them – for example shrinking them smaller or fading the colour of them? We can't delete them, but we can store them so they are less in the way some of the time.

Have you tried thinking of a place or time, recently or from a long time ago, where you felt calmer or more relaxed than you do now?

Example 3 – Grief and low mood

Bereavement and grief can present to us with wide-ranging symptoms. This case considers an approach to bereavement.

Tools

- Life raft.
- Treasure hunt (magic wand).

Patient	Anil Shah, 66 years, male.
PMH	Hypertension. Benign prostatic hypertrophy.
Medication	Doxazosin, losartan.
Social history	Lives alone. Warehouse worker.
Behaviour	Tearful, little eye contact.
Opening statement	*My boss sent me home because I might be having a breakdown.*

What do you say now?

Background

We ask some open questions and discover that, at work today, a colleague found Anil crying in the cab of his forklift. His boss suggested he might be having a breakdown and should go straight to the doctor. He would have preferred to have finished the shift. Today, he wants to talk about his physical health or just get a note for work to say that he is OK.

When we reflect – that things have been difficult recently and we ask how long things have been like this – he shares that this started about 18 months ago when his brother, to whom he was close, died unexpectedly from a stroke.

Life raft

For Anil, some topics are OK to talk about and some are difficult. Here we can use a life raft tool, as introduced in Chapter 9. This can help us balance comfortable conversations on the raft and challenging ones off it. The challenging conversations are like diving underwater, whereas, in comfortable conversations, we come up for air and rest on the raft.

First, we need to experiment to identify a safe conversation. We may choose questions needing factual answers to help Anil start talking. We watch for any topics where he volunteers extra information or seems interested or relaxes his body language.

Comfortable topics will vary: some people might be OK talking about feeling depressed and not OK talking about diabetes. For others, it may be the opposite. With Anil, we notice he enjoys talking about his workplace.

ON THE LIFE RAFT – COMFORTABLE TOPIC OR QUESTION	OFF THE LIFE RAFT – CHALLENGING QUESTIONS
How's work? What does your role involve? What do you enjoy about it?	
	Can it get stressful at work? With changes or the people there?
How long have you been there? Are there others who have been there for a similar length of time?	
	How do your friends/colleagues find the stress at work? Do they talk to each other/you? How about you? How do you cope with stressful times at work/home?
Who do you live with? Tell me about your family.	
	What do you do if you get home after a big day at work or if you are feeling stressed? How was it for your household/family when your brother died? How about you, how did you get through? How do you feel about that now?

We find out that Anil has felt very sad a lot of the time since his brother died. This is gradually lessening but today he had a sudden, huge realisation that he would never speak to his brother again. He didn't realise he was crying until his colleague banged on the window to see why he hadn't moved. He looks lost in thought and embarrassed when saying this.

We reflect that Anil is following a normal grieving process and explain,

> *Sometimes people can expect grief, the feelings and thoughts that come when someone close dies, to fit a certain timescale. What you are describing is normal, to have times when you think about your brother less and other times when you think of him and really feel his presence and absence. Different feelings are also normal – intense sadness or a fond memory.*

Information giving – grieving

We decide to explain the different facets of grief. These were first proposed by Dr Elisabath Kubler-Ross[2] as consecutive stages, but it is now thought that everyone's experience of bereavement is unique, with these happening at any time, in any order.

Shock and numbness

The numbness may be emotional – an inability to feel sad or cry or feel anything at all, or a physical feeling where skin or peripheries seem to have no sensation.

Denial

A sense that it can't be true, it must be a mistake, they must have misidentified the person, it was a "prank call", a sick joke. This cannot have happened.

Anger

Someone is at fault. A feeling of rage against the universe that has allowed this to happen or with the person who has died – *If only he had looked after himself better.*

Guilt

Maybe it was my fault. I didn't see him enough in the couple of weeks before he died. I might have been able to prevent this and now it's too late.

Bargaining

Trying to make trades or negotiating with yourself, the universe or God or a higher power to try and mitigate or undo the loss.

Depression

Intense sadness and a real longing for the person who has died. A sense of emptiness. These feelings might come and go or may be progressive, leading to depression.

Acceptance

Gradually, there comes a sense that *this is how it is now.* The person is not coming back, life will go on without them, but we can hold their presence in our hearts.

After explaining this, we decide to ask a safety question,

Some people, when someone close to them dies, have thoughts that actually dying themselves might not be a bad thing, and it might bring them closer to their loved one. These thoughts can come up for anyone. Has this ever happened to you? Tell me about that?

Anil is clear that he does not intend to end his life.

Treasure hunt – magic wand

In conversations where there is a focus on difficulties and we want to pivot towards considering the positives, we might use a magic wand question,

If we had a magic wand here now, what would you change?

Anil says he would bring his brother back, which we may have anticipated. We could follow up by asking,

What would be the first things you would do together – you and your brother?

He tells us he would hug him and tell him he loved him and how important he was to him. He would just like to spend an evening together, sitting at home doing normal things. We ask if there would be a particular conversation or something they might do. Anil says he would suggest they climb a nearby hill with views of the city. It is somewhere they used to go to remember their dad and talk about him. It was a special place, and Anil has not been there since his brother died. We reflect this,

Your brother was special enough that, when together, you could happily just enjoy each other's company. It is interesting that there is this special place for you and your brother that you haven't been to since he died.

Anil says he thinks it would feel too sad and also that he hasn't had his brother to prompt him to go there. We say,

It could be that going there brings up big emotions, and it could be somewhere that gives you a sense of calm or closeness to your brother and dad. It was important for you and your brother to remember your dad there. It can be hard when things change. Do you think you might try going again, or not so sure?

Problem-solving

We learn there have been other recent problems at work. His colleagues teased him when he cried once before, just after his brother died, and he thinks they talk to his boss about him behind his back. He hasn't done anything about this. We ask what the options might be other than doing nothing. He tells us he could go to HR, but he is not sure that would change anything other than increasing his stress. He has thought about looking for other work but fears he is too old to be considered. Despite these issues, he really enjoys working in the team and likes warehouse work. We reflect,

You enjoy your work and have a lot of experience, but you have had some issues with the workplace. You are wondering what might help and have considered going to HR or looking for other work. If you were going to take a small step towards one or both of these options, where would you start?

Anil says he has actually been looking for other work, and a next step would be to go in and speak to the team at a different warehouse. He then says that things might be no different there if he "cries like a baby" in front of a new team. We take his lead to return to this topic,

Some people might think it is not normal to show these feelings because of upbringing or what we are used to, or that it's time to move on or that you should be over it by now. But having space for these thoughts and feelings is important.

We agree on a plan with Anil. He will try returning to the hill where he used to go with his brother. He will also visit the other warehouse and talk to the team there. We offer a follow-up appointment in a couple of weeks but ensure he has a number to contact us, or a 24/7 advice line, at any time if needed. Anil says that he feels more at peace from this conversation. He says he has not really thought about it before now, but maybe it is worth going back to the hill.

Top tips for talking about problem-solving

One or more of these may be used when discussing a problem. Let's consider a situation where someone has a family event coming up and feels anxious about attending.

(Continued)

Identify and understand the problem,

> *Your cousin's birthday is next week and your family are expecting you to attend the party but you feel anxious about the number of people and some of the relationships.*

Understand options that have already been considered or tried,

> *What do you think your options are? Have you thought about any others?*

Consider strengths, expertise and experience,

> *Has there been a similar situation in the past? What did you do then? When you have this type of anxiety, what has helped you cope? When you look back, would you make the same decision?*

Ask about pros and cons,

> *What are the pros and cons of taking that option? What are the pros and cons of the other option?*

Ask about values,

> *What values are important to you? Being there for your family?*

Identify anything you have heard that could be used as a guide to plan a next step,

> *It sounds like you are leaning towards this as a way forward. Is there a small step you could try?*

References

1. Shedd, O., Sears, S., Harvill, J. et al. (2004). The World Trade Center Attack: Increased Frequency of Defibrillator Shocks for Ventricular Arrhythmias in Patients Living Remotely from New York City. J Am Coll Cardiol. 44(6):1265–7. https://doi.org/10.1016/j.jacc.2004.04.058
2. Kübler-Ross. E. (1969). On Death and Dying. The Macmillan Company.

11

Coping strategies that can cause problems

I had been using drugs and had stays as an inpatient in mental health in the past. When I went to get my certificate at the end of the course, I asked the voices *What have you got to say now?* They were silent. I had been told to "stop using" numerous times. It didn't change anything. The most success I have had in my recovery came from expanding what was good in my life. Starting with that certificate, I rebuilt my life.

Brody

Introduction

We use coping strategies when we experience stress or distress in order to tolerate, manage or even thrive physically and psychologically. They are our go-to actions or thoughts.

There are different types of coping strategies. Some may be focused on the problem,

I am too busy to walk the dog.

I'll get a dog walker and free up time to finish a work task.

DOI: 10.1201/9781003409168-14

Other strategies may focus on emotions. For example, writing an "already done list" and ticking off all the components of the work task that are complete and experiencing the positive feelings this creates.

Effective strategies will vary according to the person and their situation, so it is hard to define a "good" or "bad" strategy. Staying out late with friends chatting and debriefing may be effective after a stressful week but unhelpful the night before an exam. Factors such as our upbringing, culture and peers will also influence our own strategies.

How would I recognise a coping strategy that can cause problems?

Recreational drugs and alcohol may be perceived as potentially problematic, but the reality is more complex. Some will use these without problems. For others, 'normal activities' such as shopping or eating may become problematic. Sometimes, solutions may create a new problem – emotional, financial or affecting relationships or work. For example, paying a dog walker could add to financial stress.

Why would we use an unhelpful strategy?

Perhaps for one or more of these reasons:

- Avoidance – *It helps me avoid a thought, feeling or doing something.*
- Permission – *I can have thoughts and feelings or do something I normally wouldn't.*
- Upbringing/peers/family or cultural expectation – *Others use this strategy; perhaps I should too.*
- Pattern match – *I used this before; perhaps it will work again.*
- Short-term gain – *I will immediately feel relief/other short-term reward.*

What is self-efficacy?

"Self-efficacy" is someone's belief in their own capacity to act in ways that are needed to reach particular goals. A lack of self-efficacy may mean that a person makes self-fulfilling prophesies of failure,

I knew I couldn't stop drinking – look, I've started again. I always fail.

What can we do to support self-efficacy?

- Listen and reflect back a person's successes, however small.
- Encourage positive self-talk.
- Break down a goal or task into small, manageable, success-focused steps.
- Endorse our belief in this person's abilities.
- Support someone's recurrent attempts at tasks and stepping out of their comfort zone.
- Help plan for what to do when there are barriers or stressful times.
- Support positive social connections, including promoting links with others who have been through a similar experience and succeeded (peer support).
- Emphasise the benefits of being around people who encourage reaching for their goals.

Here, we consider three common situations where coping strategies cause, or may cause, problems:

Example 1 – Maggie Allan, 58 years. Sleep medication.

Example 2 – Kwame Green, 41 years. Alcohol use.

Example 3 – Neil Webster, 41 years. Substance use disorder.

Tools in this chapter

1 Vowels of change.
2 Add before subtract.

Additional tools

- Image or metaphor – see Chapter 5.
- What balances that? – see Chapter 9.

Vowels of change

We may use vowels (AEIOU) to help remember ways to explore the pros and cons of coping strategies.

Specific conversational tool – vowels of change

Aim	*When you use (this strategy) what are you hoping for?*
Effectiveness	*Do you find it works?*
Exceptions	*Does it ever not work?*
Increasing/decreasing.	*How often do you use (this strategy)?*
Other options	*What else do you use as well as or instead of this?*
Unwanted outcomes	*Are there any things you don't like about (this strategy)?*
Undisclosed aim	Sometimes there may be another aim which is not initially stated. It could be important to know about, e.g. smoking cannabis with the aim to relax at night; the undisclosed aim is to help anxiety present since house was broken into.

Add before subtract

If we identify a coping strategy that is causing or could cause problems, first we explore it using the vowels of change. Next, we need to ensure there are additional options in place. There may be ways to reduce the problem, or find alternative ways to cope. We discuss these new strategies before considering stopping something that is already in place.

Example 1 – sleep medication

Perhaps, the person we are talking to sees no reason to make a change, having arrived thinking, *Everything is fine, I just need a repeat prescription of something that is working.*

By contrast, the health professional, even before meeting the person, may see the potential for problems and want to make a change. The conversation will, therefore, start with little overlap in the ideas, concerns and expectations of the conversation. This is illustrated in Figure 11.1.

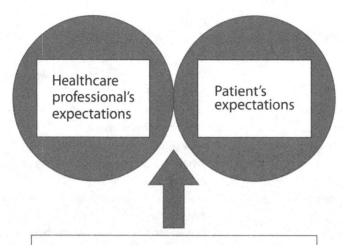

FIGURE 11.1 Healthcare professional's expectations/patient's expectations.

Here, we consider the issue of prescribed medication. We consider how to understand and explore the use of sleep medication and other approaches.

Tools

- Vowels of change.
- Add before subtract.

Patient	Maggie Allan, 58 years, female.
PMH	Depression and anxiety.
Medication	Sertraline for 15 years, zopiclone daily for last six months.
Social history	Lives with partner, works in an office. New patient – recently moved house.
Behaviour	Friendly and warm.
Opening statement	*I just want some more of the same medication the last doctors gave me. I will never be able to sleep without them.*

What do you say now?

By using open questions, we discover Maggie's ideas, concerns and expectations:

Ideas	*These tablets are great, my mood is good, I sleep well.*
Concerns	*If I stop, my mood will go back to how it was 20 years ago.*
Expectation	*Quick chat, repeat prescription*

Vowels of change

We decide to get further background information using the vowels of change,

> *It sounds like you are happy with the sleep medication. When you first started them, what difference were you hoping for?* [**A**im]

Maggie tells us she wanted a good sleep. When we probe, her aim was to fall asleep more quickly and sleep through the night. It is helpful to understand this and Maggie tells us that she used to lie awake for many hours, worrying and ruminating. She would perhaps fall asleep at 1–2 AM and be awake again around 5 AM, then get up at 7 AM.

> *Is it working? If you take the medication, do you fall asleep quickly and stay asleep?* [**E**ffectiveness]

> *Does the medication ever not work? Are there times you don't fall asleep or stay asleep?* [**E**xceptions]

Overall, Maggie is very pleased with the medication, though once, after a late conversation with her sister, she couldn't sleep and was awake most of that night.

The next two parts, I and O, consider together the reliance someone may have on this strategy and if there is any flexibility with a variety of coping strategies,

> *How often would you say you use the sleeping medication? If we went back six months ago were you using them more, or less, compared with now?* [**I**ncreasing/decreasing]

At first, she used them occasionally but now takes them most days. They work well, and her mood seems better after a good sleep,

> *Are there any nights when you have tried something else instead?*

> *What else did you try alongside the sleeping medication after the phone call with your sister?* [**O**ther options]

On this occasion, she lay awake replaying the conversation in her head. We explore this and ask,

Did you try a warm drink or relaxing shower or anything else before bed?

She says no. This is useful, as it seems to indicate the potential for other untried options. Finally, we ask whether Maggie has had any problems or side effects. [Unwanted outcomes]. She tells us – no, and no next-day drowsiness.

Exploring these has increased the overlap area in the Venn diagram. It is useful to summarise this part of the conversation, including identifying common ground,

I think we agree that sleep is important for your mental health, so it's a priority to ensure you can sleep well. The medication has helped for the last six months. Your sleep and mood have been good, and both are really important parts of health.

Uncovering an undiscovered "aim" (the reason for starting medication) can be difficult. We may explore the reasons for having a busy brain at night-time, introducing this gently with a question,

When lying awake worrying, before you had the sleeping medication, was there one particular thing or lots of different things?

Maggie tells us she had general worries, and sleep has intermittently been a problem for a long time. There was no single triggering event or specific worry.

Within a sleep consultation we would specifically explore whether it is a busy brain or busy body that is preventing sleep, and check sleep hygiene, for example avoiding caffeine and screens late in the day. We ask,

To fall asleep, we need both brain and body to be calm. Do you think your main problem with falling asleep is a busy brain or an unrelaxed body?

Maggie confirms that replaying thoughts and "busy brain" keeps her awake. We explain that our brain likes any stimulation, including worrying. It also quickly learns patterns and expects the same thing each night. This means we need to encourage our brains to be calm for us to sleep – and this can be a challenge.

Add before subtract

We move on to use the tool "add before subtract". If Maggie had identified any other options that worked for her, we could have explored these. Maggie has not given us any other options that help her sleep, but we have found out that her "busy brain" seems to keep her awake, so we decide to explore existing strategies that she may use for this,

> *If you find your brain replaying conversations like the one with your sister at other times, what do you do then? How do you manage these thoughts?*

Maggie tells us that she would watch a favourite TV show during the day, and this works well. We want to avoid screens at bedtime but could transfer the concept and see if a quiet, unexciting podcast or audio weather channel might calm her brain.

Here is a question we often use, particularly if we have not found a good strategy from the questions above,

> *Is there a time, maybe recently or some time ago, when you can remember feeling really safe and relaxed?*

Maggie doesn't respond straight away – we prompt that it could be a particular place or person, even from some time ago as a child. Her expression changes and she talks about being in her grandmother's kitchen with the smell of baking and helping prepare a meal. We ask if there was something in particular she enjoyed, and she says helping prepare the food, laughing and learning, the smells and watching the dish come together. Then we may suggest,

> *If you are in bed and you notice that your brain is becoming busy, perhaps you could try bringing up this calm memory. I can see in your face you look relaxed now, telling me about it. Maybe you can try to shrink this down and just focus on one thing, like slowly stirring a dish. We need to keep the interest level low so that our brain wants to sleep rather than continue thinking.*

In order to promote change, we suggest additional positive reasons to try something different – the advantages of change, disadvantages of not changing or both. We may give information on the limitations of sleep medication and potential side effects and suggest,

> *It may be worth having other options for sleep: there could be a time when you go away and forget the medication. Alternatively, you may find that other options work as well as the medication and it would feel good not to have the effort of regularly requesting prescriptions.*

Perhaps try thinking about being with your grandmother preparing food or having some sounds playing quietly.

Example 2 – alcohol use

This case involves a discussion about alcohol as a coping strategy.

Tools

- Vowels of change.
- Add before subtract.
- Image or metaphor.

Patient	Kwame Green, 41 years, male.
PMH	None.
Medication	None.
Social history	Divorced, 11-year-old son. Lives alone in a city flat. Works in IT.
Opening statement	*I can't hear so well in my left ear – I wondered if it was wax or something.*

What do you say now?

An alert comes up on the computer screen mid-consultation – it is nearly the year-end and, in order to reach a target and financial reward, the practice urgently needs to record more patients' alcohol consumption and offer a brief intervention if appropriate.

We have had a straightforward consultation and confirmed there is wax. As we have time, we decide to ask about alcohol. We find that Kwame and his work colleagues are very sociable and go out drinking every Friday. Team building days also involve alcohol. Most evenings, he drinks at home.

We use the vowels of change.

Aim

Sometimes we do things through habit, other times because they help with something. Tell me about drinking alcohol at the end of every day.

After a stressful day, this is Kwame's highlight: the sip of cold beer instantly creates a feeling of relaxation.

Effectiveness and exceptions

Would you say it works? If the aim is to relax, does it relax you?

Are there any times you have got home, had some beer and not had that relief and relaxation?

Kwame tells us it usually works, though there was a time recently arguing with his ex-wife over his son when he still felt really stressed despite alcohol. We may want to explore this more but first we continue with the vowels of change.

Increasing/decreasing

Over time would you say you are increasing or decreasing your alcohol intake, or is it about the same?

Kwame says he totally stopped drinking alcohol when his son was born but, since his marriage ended, he has been drinking again for the last year or so.

Other options

If you want to relax, what other things help, as well as or instead of alcohol?

When you're at work or feeling stressed from speaking to your ex, what do you try?

Every other weekend, he feels relaxed and happy when he is with his son. At work he is distracted by tasks and being around others. We reflect that the social side of being around other people is, perhaps, relaxing. At home, in the evenings, he typically drinks alone.

We ask about socialising outside of work and he tells us he has always been a social person but having moved house he has lost contact with many friends.

Unwanted effects

Is there anything you don't like about drinking alcohol? What would be your main reasons for thinking about reducing alcohol?

He tells us just to improve his general health. We can hold this up to a "truth light". Is this meaningful? Is he really interested in improving his health or is it a "textbook" answer? It doesn't seem like a big motivation for him to change.

Undisclosed aims

Is he using alcohol to avoid a thought or feeling or something he should be doing? We summarise,

> *I'm hearing that alcohol is in your life now more than in the past, and even though you think reducing it would be good for your general health, it is one of the few things that is helping you relax in the evenings, with the changes from your marriage ending. You use it to relax and it helps.*

> *If you got home and didn't drink a beer, what would you do or think about?*

Kwame tells us that he might cry. He tells us how much he misses his son. He finds it hard to think of him or look at his photo without feeling overwhelmed with emotion. He feels guilty and that he is letting his son down. He is on the brink of tears talking about this. We acknowledge this additional aim and then repeat the vowels of change to incorporate this newly disclosed aim,

> *You are a devoted father and live for the time you can spend with your son. It is incredibly difficult for you to be apart and, when you are home alone in the evening, you focus on drinking alcohol rather than the guilt and sadness of not being with your son.*

Now we can ask if alcohol works for this aim,

> *Does it work? Do you find drinking alcohol helps, so you feel less guilty or not as sad?*

Kwame tells us he doesn't think about it as much, but it is always in his head. Last week there was one occasion when he was both drinking and crying. We reflect this,

> *On that day, alcohol – in some ways – gave you permission to let out the grief and sadness you have been feeling.*

We can move to other options,

> *If you think about your son and start to feel sad, perhaps guilty, are there other things you can do that might help with those thoughts and feelings?*

Kwame avoids these thoughts and feelings where possible and is unsure what helps. We reflect that being at work, around others and focusing on tasks, help to distract him. We return to ask about unwanted consequences,

> *Have there been times alcohol has got in the way of you enjoying time with your son?*

He tells us there haven't.

We have defined the problem, but we can't increase his contact with his son, so what can we do?

What balances that?

We now understand that the aim of alcohol use is to avoid feelings but also to give permission to think about his son and feel a range of emotions. The gap is with alternatives, so we use the "what balances that?" tool,

> *If you are sitting with a beer and thinking about your son, you tend to think about the negatives, like feeling guilty and sad. What is a fond, positive memory that balances that?*

Kwame tells us about teaching his son to ride his bike last weekend. We want to affirm this,

> *You and your son create some amazing memories on alternate weekends. You are a caring and protective person in his life.*

If, one evening, you wanted to think about a positive memory of your son like that, what would remind you?

Kwame says maybe looking at photos or videos on his phone. But he avoids this because he starts to feel angry with his ex-wife and doesn't want to get caught up in that or cry.

Image or metaphor

We might reflect using a metaphor to say,

> *A rope formed of intertwined strands is stronger. In the same way, the intertwined happy and sad thoughts can make a strong connection between you and your son regardless of distance. It might be helpful to let the positive and negative thoughts intertwine.*

This reframe may give him a different perspective on emotions that he may have been taught to avoid or hide – guilt, anger, shame. Now we might introduce the idea of subtracting alcohol,

If you had times when it felt OK to think about your son and feel all those feelings – happiness, sadness, anger, grief, guilt and caring, protective love – and if you didn't need the beer, what else might you do in the evening?

Kwame tells us he probably needs to consider more permanent housing: a longer lease or buying somewhere; perhaps put down roots and join a sports team. He has thought about dating again. We reflect on what he has told us and link in values to help inspire him to take action,

It sounds as if life has been on hold for a bit. Maybe the habit of drinking alcohol has been part of that, and you got into a bit of a rut. When you step back and look at what you enjoy and how you want to be, you have been considering changing things. Maybe now is a good time to take the next step. Perhaps these thoughts about settled housing and joining a sports team are helping you understand the type of role model you want to be for your son.

Kwame agrees that he would like to explore joining a sports team. Perhaps his son would enjoy coming to training or matches. Housing is his second priority. We agree a specific, achievable plan and time frame and the consultation ends with agreement for a phone review in four weeks.

Add before subtract

Problem X (anxiety since house break-in) = Solution A (use cannabis)

If we suggest removing solution A, i.e. stop using cannabis, this is less likely to be successful than if we understand the problem and ensure there are other options for solutions first.

Problem X (anxiety since house break-in) = Solution A (use cannabis) +/– Solution B (listen to a podcast) +/– Solution C (breathing exercises)

Example 3 – substance use disorder

Recovery from a substance use disorder is not a single pass/fail event. It is a chronic condition and recovery occurs over time. How do we best support this in primary care? When making a change is difficult, we consider whether the person who will make the change can answer these questions,

What is my motivation to change? Why should I?

Do I believe I am able to make the change? Can I?

The second part of these questions refers to self-efficacy. Higher self-efficacy means we are more likely to achieve our goals, even when we encounter stresses or barriers, and is associated with addiction recovery. An indication of low self-efficacy is when you hear a patient expressing self-fulfilling failure, *There is no point in trying, I will never succeed.* This could be an indication to involve a wider team. In this case we consider how we in primary care can support building someone's self-efficacy.

Tools

- Add before subtract,
- What balances that?
- Image or metaphor – rulebook/hands.

Patient	Neil Webster, 35 years, male.
PMH	Notes from local drug/alcohol service four years ago. Bloods 18 months ago – HIV and hepatitis negative.
Medication	None.
Social history	Lives in temporary housing.
Expectations	Cream for rash. Don't want a lecture.
Opening statement	*I am just here to sort out this rash, not for anything else.*

What do you say now?

Background

There is visible eczema and scratch marks on his forearms and legs. After discussing this, we decide to consider Neil's overall health, including mental health and substance use disorder.

Add before subtract

First, we want to find out what is currently good about life and how, ideally, Neil would like things to improve. We open this conversation with a "zoom-out" open question,

Thinking overall about your health and life, what is going well for you? Which areas of life are better than others at the moment?

Neil tells us that, recently, he nearly became homeless again but managed to find temporary housing. We ask how he achieved this. He knew about this accommodation through a friend who had stayed there and contacted the place directly. We reflect this and include the positives we have heard,

That was quite a close thing, finding housing in time, and it was because you prioritised this and because of your social connections that it worked out. It was good you thought of contacting your friend and that you spoke up for yourself with the accommodation.

Neil says he would like to sort out his housing. We hear he has been moving frequently, staying in temporary accommodation and sometimes being kicked out due to drug use.

Magic wand question

Moving frequently is hard. If you had a magic wand, what would your housing situation be like?

Neil tells us he would just like to have somewhere to rent where he knew he could stay and set up a home. We ask,

Have you had times in the past recently, or long ago, where you have been able to put down roots or had somewhere that has felt like home?

Neil lived with his brother for five years and that felt like home. They would eat together in the evenings and talk. He is no longer in contact with his brother after problems that arose through Neil's drug use. He says, *That's what I do, ruin everything.* We reframe this and continue to focus on the positives. First, we zoom in,

When we look back, we sometimes judge ourselves harshly, but perhaps we can learn what's important to us from things that went wrong or felt "ruined". Maybe this has helped you realise that you really want a home. I wonder if you are also being self-critical because your brother is important to you. When you have somewhere permanent, what will you do first to make it "home"?

Neil says he would like to get some houseplants, as these always make him feel homely. Growing up, his parents had plants around the house. We ask if he has ever had plants or a garden himself. He looked after his brother's but hasn't since then. We ask,

Is that something you are considering? Have you thought about which plant you might get?

Neil says it's pointless. He is resigned to his life going around the same circles and not getting accommodation. We reflect, using the values that Neil has shared,

> *It can be hard to stay motivated, particularly when things feel tougher than we would like, but you are keen to have somewhere to call "home". When you do, that might also be a step towards more evenings sitting and chatting with your brother, but this time at your home.*

What balances that?

Neil agrees but says it won't work out. We decide to use the "What balances that?" tool and ask,

> *We all have times when a negative voice tells us things like, "There is no point in trying". What is the opposite thought? Do you have something positive you tell yourself to balance these negatives?*

Neil cannot think of anything. We ask,

> *Can you think of anyone recently, or maybe longer ago, who spoke to you in an encouraging way, maybe someone who believed in you?*

Neil tells us that his teacher did when he was 13-years-old. We ask what they might say if they were here now and still encouraging him. He says they would tell him, "Keep going, you will get there, Neil". We might re-enforce this as a strategy,

> *How does it feel now to hear, "Keep going, you will get there, Neil?" That sounds like a helpful thought and could balance, "There's no point". Do you think that is something you could say to yourself?*

Another step would be to harness Neil's strengths from the recent housing difficulty and see if these could be transferred to future situations,

> *Wanting a roof over your head recently, you had a vision and stayed focused. You didn't notice the "what's the point" voice, and it didn't stop you from doing what you wanted.*

Image or metaphor

We might use a metaphor; one we think Neil might relate to: the idea of "breaking rules",

Perhaps thinking "What's the point" and "I will fail" has become the rule-book. You ignored this and broke the rule when you decided to sort out your housing. Maybe you have started to work on a new rulebook and not listen to some of these old rules.

We end the conversation and give Neil the prescription for his eczema and offer to see him again any time he would like to discuss things further.

Top tips talking about addictions[1]

- Ask about the 4Cs (compulsions, cravings, consequences, control) aiming to identify addiction early because prompt intervention can reduce the time to remission.
- Provide support for the journey – addiction recovery is not one pass/fail event, nor is the pathway linear. Treat it as a chronic condition and accept unforeseen recurrence as part of the path to recovery. "Remission" is at five years when the risk of relapse is the same as in the general population. Continue support to this point.
- There is research showing the benefit of being involved in mutual-help groups such as Alcoholics Anonymous (AA). It is worth encouraging these in conversations.
- Consider having conversations where the focus is a nudge *towards* a desired future or goal instead of a focus on pushing away from an undesired coping strategy.
- When deciding a next step, start small and strength-based. Consider self-efficacy and, if needed, make the step smaller to increase the likelihood of success

Reference

1. https://www.recoveryanswers.org/ [accessed 5 May, 2023].

12

Conversations when there is not much time

These are really important conversations. Sometimes it felt like there was all this interest in whether I was suicidal, but unless I was, or met some other invisible target, I was offered nothing. I felt like I wasn't good enough at being depressed.

Jane Fausett

Introduction

And while I'm here…

Insufficient time and inadequate tools make for a perfect storm – an unsatisfactory consultation for both clinician and patient. With little time left, we may often use our interpersonal and communication skills to simply rebook another appointment. But, in this chapter, we consider whether there are ways to give people a new perspective or takeaway tool even within a very brief conversation. We also consider ways to manage some common *and while I'm here* questions.

We will look at three patients who challenge us by presenting significant problems when we have little time left in the consultation:

Example 1 – May Lee, 33 years. Crying when there are two minutes left.

Example 2 – Winston Hall, 56 years. Unspecified mental health concern.

Example 3 – Yusuf Akhtar, 41 years. *I'm just wondering whether it is worth going on.*

DOI: 10.1201/9781003409168-15

Tools in this chapter

- Better–worse.

This tool is used to deepen our understanding initially without finding a specific situation to discuss. These general comparison questions can help to identify a specific situation, which can be easier to discuss.

Are there times when you feel better and worse?

What would you be out of 10 right now?

Is there a time when you felt worse than this?

Additional tools

- HOLLA 321 – see Chapter 1.
- Metaphor – see Chapter 5.
- Coping questions – see Chapter 6.
- Think, feel, do (body and you) – see Chapter 6.
- Choose the focus – see Chapter 7.

Example 1 – crying when there are two minutes left

Here, we use a metaphor to approach the situation of someone displaying a big emotion, for example, crying, when we have very little time left for this conversation.

Tools

- Image or metaphor – ride the wave
- Choose the focus
- Coping questions.

Patient	May Lee, 33 years, female.
PMH	Nothing of note.
Social history	Lives with partner, works as a waitress.
Behaviour	Quiet.
Opening statement	*My periods are really heavy – is there anything I can take?*

Background

We have had an uneventful consultation with May about her periods, including the next steps and management. There are a couple of minutes left, and we are just wrapping up when May starts to cry. She has been relatively quiet in the consultation, but this is unexpected.

How can we help and make the best use of the remaining time?

Image or metaphor – ride the wave

We use the idea of being at sea and the emotion hitting both of us in the conversation like a big, perhaps unexpected, wave.

Firstly, we have to choose which direction to take. We could go towards the emotion and explore it. This is like moving out into the waves. We might use minimal encouragers and non-verbal prompts to encourage May to stay with her feelings and perhaps continue to cry. If we choose this, we might use a tool like "think, feel, do" and ask, *What thoughts are going through your head now?*

The second option is to move the conversation away from this emotion and towards the shore, a more certain destination. We may decide to do this at the outset, or we may first explore the emotion and waves but then guide us both back to shore. How do we do this?

Ride the wave (choose the focus)

We use the "choose the focus" tool. First, we need to re-engage with May, bringing her out of her strong emotions and back in the room with us by using words to guide her out of her feelings, memories and thoughts. We use our tone and volume to convey that the situation, even with this emotion, is safe and manageable.

Trying to bring the focus back to the present, we may start speaking even over the crying, starting with a soft tone of voice at a quieter, slower pace and then gradually bringing the volume and pace of speech towards normal. We may choose one of the following.

"Ride the wave" comments

There's a lot going on. You have had to be strong.

It seems like things have been building for a while.

I'm not surprised there are moments when there are tears.

There's a lot going on emotionally for you.

It can be hard to give time for these emotions.

It can take strength to let tears out/really show how you are feeling.

Opening up like this can take courage.

The message running through all these statements is,

> *Things have been tough, but you are strong.*

As with all suggestions, be authentic and find words that work for you. Note that we do not label the tears with an emotion, e.g. *You are sad,* as we do not yet know if these tears are due to sadness, guilt, embarrassment or any other emotion.

Switch tools (coping questions)

We look for signs that the person's attention is back in the room with us. Perhaps they are making some or more eye contact, or the volume or amount of crying may have changed. We know we are heading for the shore.

Once we notice that someone is now present, we want to quickly make a "switch" towards dry land and away from the sea.

The switch entails moving away from thinking about thoughts, feelings and worries, instead looking towards strengths and ways of coping that are helpful. We can perhaps think of the image of standing on a surfboard and jumping from facing one way to facing the other.

We might introduce the switch by validating the emotion and then asking a coping question. We say to May,

> *It seems to me that there have been some tough times for you. It looked like there was a lot going through your mind. Crying can be important; we often don't make time for these big emotions. With all the things that have been happening that you were thinking about just now, what are the ways you have been coping with everything?*

How this question is phrased is important. The message we are aiming to convey is that there are ways that May **has** been coping with everything, however difficult. This is different from asking, *How have you been coping?*, which is likely to be answered with *I haven't* or *I don't know...*, which does not help us identify strengths and strategies. However, even with this phrasing, May tells us she is not coping. We may need to ask coping questions twice and follow up by saying,

> *It sounds really hard. What do you think has been helping you get through the day?*

May tells us that meditating helps her to feel calm and present in the moment.

Switch using treasure hunt questions

Alternatively, if May had still struggled to answer this, we might use a treasure hunt question,

> *If we think about all the thoughts that are behind these tears, all that is going on for you, what are you doing differently day-to-day?*

This may be a hard question to answer, and we may need to de-code the answer. Let's say May tells us that nothing is different, and she has to go to work and keep up her routine. She finds herself distracted and was relieved not to get in trouble for being late to a work meeting and forgetting some paperwork. We could reflect this and include a switch to try and get an answer to the same question,

> *At the moment, there are times when you are caught up in your thoughts. When was a time when you were really present in the moment and very much involved in something you were doing?*

May tells us she is Buddhist and when she is meditating, she feels calm and present. Also, sometimes at work she will be able to focus on a task but can feel distracted in meetings and find it harder to concentrate. We might check whether there has been any change in how often she meditates and may use this as part of a plan.

Next step plan, follow-up and safety

After discussing coping tools, we can now face the waves but have a little more distance between us and them,

There has been a lot on your mind lately, and taking time to meditate is something that gives you some calm in the day. These are useful skills and something that is important to continue. When we are busy, we might stop prioritising things that keep us healthy and functioning when we need them more than ever.

We could also offer the opportunity to fully face the waves and explore what is behind the crying,

I know there is a lot we haven't discussed today. I wonder if it would be useful for us to make time to talk again?

Safety

In a conversation like this, which has been very brief, we would always want to touch on safety,

It seems to me that things have been tough, and I would like to check that you feel safe. When you leave here today, do you have any concerns for your safety? That you might be at risk? Either from something you might do or from anyone else?

May tells us she is not concerned about her safety and that she will rebook to come back. She suggests in a month, but we suggest sooner, for example next week, but we will let her decide. We end with a summary and backup plan. As we have not explored the emotion, it is important that we ensure that there is permission to explore this in the future. We say,

I'm really pleased you felt able to share these feelings today. I think you showed what a strong person you are. I also think meditating helps you cope with difficult times, and it is worth prioritising doing this daily. If you have times when you feel things are worse or it is hard to cope, then please get back in touch with the practice, and here is the number for a 24/7 support line.

Example 2 – unspecified mental health concern

Here, we consider an undifferentiated mental health problem that has come up just when we thought the conversation was closing. We are not sure what the symptom or potential diagnosis might be.

Sometimes, even after asking relevant questions, it is unclear how and why someone's mental health is being affected. If it is not quickly apparent that there has been a stressful event (relationship ending, loss of work, previous trauma) or specific symptoms, then there can be additional complexity. This example provides an approach to this situation.

Tools

- Better–worse.
- Think, feel, do (body and you).
- Coping questions based on "think, feel, do (body and you)".

Patient	Winston Hall, 56 years, male.
PMH	Gout.
Social history	Single. Civil engineer.
Behaviour	Normal, appears mentally well.
Opening statement	*It's my gout again. Can I get some of those tablets that helped before?*

The consultation about gout is complete. With two minutes left, as the conversation is wrapping up, he says,

And I think I need to sort out my mental health.

How can we approach this?

Background

It might feel preferable to postpone this conversation for a further visit, but we can use our remaining time to find out more and ensure that Winston is safe.

Better–worse

We use the better-worse tool to start with generalisations:

I'm wondering if there are times when you feel better and other times when you feel worse.

What would you be out of 10 right now?

Is there a time when you felt worse than you do now?

Winston tells us that he felt worse last week at work. We have used general questions to get to a specific situation and can then ask more about how he felt on this occasion. He tells us he was working at a building site, feeling increasingly anxious and wanting to escape.

Think, feel, do (body and you)

> *At that time, did you have particular thoughts or memories?* (These don't have to be disclosed.)

> *And when you had those thoughts/memories did you notice anything happening with your body? Maybe your heart racing or feeling sweaty?*

Winston says his stomach was churning, so we ask,

> *What was the feeling that went with those thoughts or memories when your stomach was churning? And what was going through your head when you were wanting to escape?*

Typically, people answer questions about feelings by telling us about thoughts or actions, e.g. *I thought about calling an ambulance.*

This thought can then be reflected in order to find the feeling,

> *How did it feel having your stomach churning so much that you thought you might need to call an ambulance?*

Now we get to the feeling, *Frightening, I was scared.*

Winston identifies that his stomach often churns, and he feels nauseous and scared. It is worse when he visits his mother, who is in a hospice, or sees his sister, who is normally supportive but with whom he recently argued. He feels as if he can't cope and is worried about his future relationship with his sister. We help Winston connect his thoughts and feelings with the symptoms he experiences, and his actions.

We can now move to the next step and ask…

Coping questions based on think, feel, do (body and you)

> *When you get that feeling, what do you do?*

> *What helps you when you feel like that?*

What feeling would help – what could you add to balance feeling scared?

What things do you do when you feel safe?

The conversation naturally carries on to revisit each of the "think, feel, do (body and you)" responses to identify ways to cope from a mental health perspective. It could be that only one question is needed to find a couple of good coping strategies that can be continued until the next, fuller, conversation.

Winston tells us he drinks moderate amounts of alcohol to cope. He would like to feel more relaxed. Usually, he feels this way with his sister and her family and has memories of family beach holidays. He also enjoys socialising with friends but has not seen them recently. Reflecting this back to Winston, we make a plan. He will look through some holiday photos, contact his adult nephew and arrange a time to see friends this week.

This brief conversation concludes with a safety question and plan for follow-up,

In terms of wanting to sort your mental health, does this feel OK as a first step? Do you feel safe with this plan? Let's meet again to see how things are, and in the meantime, what will you do if you feel really bad or not safe?

Winston says he feels safe and agrees to try this plan. He could contact his sister, day or night, and knows she would answer. We provide a 24/7 contact number for advice and help.

Specific conversational tool – think, feel, do (body and you)

"Think, feel, do" uses the elements from a CBT five-part model.[1] It is a way of "zooming in" to understand a problem. It works on the premise that each of these categories is closely linked. Changing one – for example an action – can change the others (thoughts, feelings, physiology).

We might phrase this as a previous event, *When you were out inspecting the site...*, or a generalisation including past and future, *When you are at site inspections....* Typically, we would start using this tool by asking a question that lets the person choose which area to answer first,

When you are at the site, what do you notice happening in your body – or is there a particular thought or feeling?

(Continued)

Next, we can ask more about this same category or we can move to ask about another category. Sometimes we may ask generally and let the person choose,

> *What else do you notice?*

Then we would move through each remaining area,

Think: *When you turned around as if to leave, what thoughts went through your head?*

Feel: *What emotions did (might) you notice?*

Do: *What did you notice in your body? What was the first thing you did when you had this thought that you wanted to leave?*

We would demonstrate the links between these in a summary.

The next step could be to consider general strategies, for example by zooming out with a coping question. Or we may work within the model by planning to do something differently to see if it changes the other interlinked areas,

> *The idea of taking a deep breath and thinking about holidays together at the beach could be worth trying to see what difference it makes to how you feel.*

Example 3 – *I just wonder whether it is worth going on*

Here, we focus on developing a safety plan at the end of the conversation when there is little time left.

Tool

- HOLLA 321.

Patient	Yusuf Akhtar, 41 years, male.
PMH	Type 2 diabetes.
Medication	Metformin.
Social history	Married with three children. Solicitor.
Behaviour	Slightly anxious.
Opening statement	*I've had this pain in my knee after running for the last two weeks.*

Background

We have had a straightforward musculoskeletal consultation about the knee pain and briefly checked his diabetes control and that he has a nurse review appointment. He has hinted a couple of times that work is stressful, and that he is under pressure. We have sympathised but not explored this. The consultation is wrapping up, and Yusuf is standing near the door and says,

I sometimes wonder if it's all worth it, you know?

Do we need to respond at all? Would asking anything further mean another 10 minutes of conversation?

We **must** respond! It is essential to follow up all comments that indicate a patient may be at risk of self-harm, however casual they may seem.

Clarifying

First, we need to clarify what Yusuf means. Is he talking about a change of career or is he hinting at thoughts of ending his life?

Yeah, I know. What do you mean when you say you wonder if it's "worth it"?

Yusef responds vaguely, saying sometimes everything feels a bit much, and he goes on to tell us it's nothing and turns towards the door. We further clarify, watching closely for how Yusuf responds,

At times when things feel overwhelming and "everything feels a bit much", it is common to have thoughts like, "Would it be better to go to sleep and not wake up?" Is that what you meant when you said, "Is it worth going on?"

Yusuf confirms this is what he meant, and we explore whether he has ever made any specific plans or taken any action either recently or in the past. He clearly and congruently says not; it has only been a thought. He seems uncomfortable discussing this much further. Alongside our clinical judgement, we go on to use the following brief approach,

Is it OK to just talk briefly about this for a minute or so before you go? It's not uncommon to think like this when we are stressed and it can be worth having a quick plan.

Yusuf has turned back towards us, so we continue.

HOLLA 321 – one-minute safety check

Having confirmed that someone has made an in-passing or parting comment about thoughts of ending their life, we could use this one-minute approach: 3 questions, 2 strategies, 1 person – HOLLA.

Three questions – HOLLA (*How Often? Long Lasting? Act?*)

We want to deepen our understanding of the situation by asking three questions:

1 Frequency – *How often are you thinking these types of thoughts?*
2 Lasting – *Do the thoughts come into your head and go again quickly, or do they stick around?*
3 Act – *Do they bother you? Have you ever acted on these thoughts? Do you think you ever would?*

Here is how we might structure the conversation,

How often would you say you are having these thoughts? Many times a day or only now and then?

OK, perhaps twice in the last few weeks. And when those thoughts came into your head, did they come and just go again, or did they stick around and maybe you started thinking more about them?

It sounds as if they stayed quite briefly. How much did it bother you to have these thoughts?

Yusuf was concerned. He had never had thoughts like this come into his head before and does feel anxious about if they came back. We clarify whether this affected him at the time or afterwards,

At the time when you had this thought, did you feel safe? Did you think you might do something?

Yusuf tells us he was not worried about his safety on either of these occasions. He has never taken any action and would never end his life. He just doesn't understand why he thought it at all. He is concerned that the thought might come back, though he thinks it is unlikely, as he has recently met a work deadline.

Two strategies

Now, we look to the future and the possibility of this thought returning. We want to know Yusuf's plan – at least two options – for how to feel safe even with this thought,

> *If this happens again, what will you do to cope while this thought is in your brain?*

Yusuf is not sure how to answer this. We ask what he did the last time he had this thought, in order to look for the current coping approaches he is using. He tells us he was in bed, and he thought about his family and an event that weekend that he was expecting his wife and children to enjoy. We rephrase this back,

> *Thinking about people who are important to you seemed to work well. If you left here and your brain suddenly came up with the thought, "Is it all worth it?" would you use this again? Is there anything else you might try if this thought was sticking around, something that would help you cope – and feel safe – while this thought was there?*

Yusuf tells us the other time it happened was at work when he was given some extra, unexpected work. He got up and walked out of the building. We reflect this – that perhaps physically moving around, changing place and noticing different things outside may have helped.

One person

We would ideally like at least one other person to be aware and involved or an option for contacting at least one service at any time. We ask Yusuf,

> *If these thoughts of "Is it worth it?" come up, you could try some of these options, perhaps thinking of things and people important to you or moving around or changing where you physically are. If you still had these thoughts and they were bothering you, who would you talk to?*

Yusuf looks shocked and says he does not want his family to know. He doesn't think this situation would happen. We reflect that sometimes it can be easier to talk to someone we don't know. We ask,

> *If there was a situation where you needed to involve someone else in order to feel safe, who would you contact?*

Yusuf would not want to speak to anyone he knew. He would find it easier to use an anonymous helpline as a backup.

Summary

Finally, we might summarise,

> We all have times when we are stressed, and our brains come up with thoughts we wouldn't have at other times. That can include thoughts like "Is it worth it?" and "Would it be better if I wasn't here?" The ways of coping you have already used – thinking about things/people important to you, moving around or going somewhere else – seem to be working. If these don't work, if you are concerned about those thoughts, let me know, or you can contact this crisis 24/7 number.

More thoughts, more people

Depending on how often and persistent these thoughts are, how much they are troubling someone, and the strategies they have in place for managing thoughts of self-harm, we may want to involve a wider team and ask,

> Does anyone else know about you having these types of thoughts?

> Who would you tell? How would you contact them?

> Do they feel worried about your safety? What might they do?

> How could they best help keep you safe?

We might normalise here – particularly around it being common to feel that sharing this would burden others. Then we balance that with whether those close to us may have noticed or be worrying already. Sharing this problem together may be a relief for both people, to support each other. We may decide that the safest option is to involve more people before ending the conversation, with a joint call or contact from Yusuf to a friend or relative or, if needed, involving additional health services.

HOLLA 321

We can use this framework to start conversations where we might otherwise be tempted to ignore a passing comment. It does not replace usual clinical management and, where needed to ensure safety, usual pathways should be followed.

Top tips – ending the conversation

At the end of a mental health conversation there are some important tasks to complete.

1. **Lock in the next step(s)**
   Consider identifying:
   - Something that will be continued that is already a **habit**.
   - Something to restart, or something new to start – if there is strong motivation and it is likely to be achievable.
   - Something that is a **maybe** to consider.

     Habit – *It sounds like you will continue your usual walking, three days a week.*

     Likely – *You are keen to spend more time with your adult children, so will phone both your sons this week.*

     Maybe – *You might start looking into a creative writing course.*

2. **Agree when to talk again**
   Think about the practicalities. Will the next step be with you or someone else? If a different team member, discuss this before the person leaves.

     How shall we check in to see how you are?

     Is a phone call better or face-to-face?

     I work closely with the team here; can I arrange for (named role/ person) to call you? Is this the best number for you?

3. **Make sure there is a backup plan**

     In the meantime, if you have any times when it would help to talk or you feel worse, get in touch sooner, or you can call this number 24/7 to get support.

Thinking particularly about safety, we might check who else could be involved,

If we have trouble contacting you, is there someone else you are OK with us talking to – who/what number? If we did end up talking to them, what would you be OK with and what would you definitely not want us to share?

Reference

1. Padesky, C.A., & Mooney, K.A. (1990). Presenting the Cognitive Model to Clients. Int J Cogn Ther. 6:13–4. Available at www.padesky.com

13

Conversations when there is a context of trauma

I had never been able to have a smear test. I saw that it said there were staff with an interest in anxiety and mental health. They used breathing and other techniques with me – I was so proud to get my smear!

Pooja*

Introduction

Sometimes, we encounter people who have experienced trauma, whether in the past or recently, and this may continue to affect them. Trauma can take different forms – from a person who experienced abuse as a child, a woman who is experiencing coercive controlling behaviour now, or the physical and emotional trauma of a recent serious road traffic incident.

It is important to recognise that having one or many experiences of trauma does not mean that a person will have problems with mental health. Many people with experience of trauma do not have anxiety, low mood or any emotional problems. But trauma can mean that someone reacts with big emotions to small situations or uses coping strategies that can cause problems such as problems with alcohol, drugs or self-harm, and there is an association between trauma and some mental health problems – post-traumatic stress disorder (PTSD), anxiety and depression.

DOI: 10.1201/9781003409168-16

When we suspect trauma, whether or not we overtly discuss it, we take care to use trauma-informed approaches. We ensure that the physical environment is safe, that we behave in a clear and collaborative way, and that people have choices.

In this chapter, we will look at three different presentations of trauma in primary care:

Example 1 – Mandy Howard, 57, female. Nightmares, flashbacks and anxiety.

Example 2 – Imani McFarlane, 20, female. Suicide attempt/discharged from A&E.

Example 3 – Anthony Evans, 43, male. Overwhelming emotion, anger.

Tools in this chapter

1 Self-compassion.
2 ABC – antecedents, behaviour, consequences.

Additional tools

- Image or metaphor – TV, broken radio, storm – see Chapter 5.
- What balances that? – see Chapter 9.
- Shrink it – see Chapter 10.

Self-compassion

Self-compassion means responding to ourselves with kindness, particularly when we fail, suffer or feel inadequate, and recognising that we are all imperfect and that this is part of being human. It helps create feelings of safety and contentment. Increased self-compassion can help many mental health symptoms.

ABC – antecedents, behaviour, consequences

The ABC psychological model enables us to find out what happened before a particular event, for example an overdose of paracetamol:

- **Antecedents** – *Before X, what were you thinking and feeling? What did you do? Was there a particular trigger that finally tipped you to X?*

- **Behaviour** – *Actions – When you were deciding to X did you consider any other actions? At that moment, did you have a particular outcome that you wanted?*
- **Consequences** – "Next and now" – *What happened straight after you X? What were you thinking and feeling and what did you do? How do you feel now, looking back? What would you say are the pros and cons of this action?*

Example 1 – nightmares, flashbacks and anxiety

Here, we introduce the idea of using a trauma-informed approach where we ensure equity of power between clinician and patient and check that we have consent to continue rather than assuming an automatic right to ask questions and probe previous traumatic events.

Tools

- Image or metaphor – TV.
- Self-compassion.

Patient	Mandy Howard, 57 years, female.
PMH	Recent road traffic accident – checked out at A&E – no problems, discharged. Fit note for two weeks.
Social history	Lives alone. Work – chain restaurant, office role.
Behaviour	Quiet, nervous, on edge.

On your task list today is the following message: *"Mandy Howard requests further fit note – still not right after the car crash".*

What do you do now?

Background

The notes show recent trauma – the car crash – but we don't know whether there are physical or psychological problems, or a mix, making Mandy feel "not right". We decide to work in a trauma-informed way – with regular consent and giving choices so she feels in control. We phone and start with an introduction and options of who to talk to and when,

I think you got in touch about extending your fit note. Are you OK to talk with me now, over the phone? Alternatively, I or one of my colleagues could call at a different time, or we could arrange to meet in person. What works best for you?

Then, we either negotiate an appointment or, if we get a go-ahead, cover confidentiality and who to involve or not. In a phone conversation, this step is particularly important,

I am here on my own, and everything we talk about will be treated confidentially like all health information. May I ask, are you on your own or with anyone else? Do you want us to include anyone else at this point?

Mandy describes nightmares and feeling anxious since a car accident on a country road in the dark two weeks ago. She was hit from behind. The driver got out briefly, smelling of alcohol, and promptly left. Her car was damaged but driveable. She went to A&E and was checked out – nothing serious; her neck and muscle aches are slowly improving. She often works late evenings, and now even thinking about driving in the dark makes her feel panicky. She is, therefore, hoping for more time off work.

She has driven once in the daytime since the accident – to the supermarket – and felt anxious throughout. She has not been back to work. She gets flashbacks of the crash and feels she is reliving it.

Metaphor – TV

We move into management by acknowledging what she has told us and then sharing an image, taken from ACT, to try to start to reduce the intensity of the feelings – again being careful with consent and empowering the patient,

Can I explain what I'm hearing – and because we can't see each other, anytime you want me to pause or it feels unhelpful, could you say "pause" or "hey", or hang up and I can call back. That would be helpful for me. Will that work for you? Can you do a "hey" just so I can check I can hear? Thanks.

Experiencing flashbacks is normal after a traumatic event and, mostly, this lessens over time. Right now, when you notice feeling panicky and relive what happened, it's as if you are in a cinema. The image of the crash is on a huge wraparound screen. The surround sound is booming. It might feel like it is closing in on you.

I'd like you to try watching the image back again, but this time turning the volume down so low it is barely possible to hear, shrinking the picture from a movie screen right down to a tiny watch screen. Vivid colours become muted shades of grey.

If you think about something from the flashback in this way, does it feel any different? Does it feel easier and less overwhelming? Sometimes shrinking the images and sounds like this can change how it feels.

If Mandy finds it hard to keep the screen small, we can suggest tools to help keep her "present" in the here and now rather than stuck in the trauma cinema,

Notice something near and something far.

Count the number of times you can see a particular colour.

Feel the texture of your clothing.

We make a plan to try this out and speak again soon about a return to work. This might include an activity ladder – e.g. a phased return, initially travelling only during daylight hours.

Acute trauma on a background of previous trauma

Mandy's relatively minor RTA has triggered symptoms that we might find with post-traumatic stress disorder (PTSD). If, at further reviews, she still has ongoing anxiety or other symptoms, we might wonder whether there has been previous trauma. We might ask a general question,

After this experience, how are you feeling now about life overall?

We may follow up more specifically, perhaps with statements used as questions, to take the pressure off the need for her to answer,

I am wondering if this experience has made you look at your life differently in any way.

Sometimes when we experience a big event like this, it can make us step back and think about life overall.

We may ask more specifically while seeking consent as we introduce a new topic,

You don't have to answer this, and it may not be relevant to you, but sometimes an event like this can bring up memories from other big events that have happened over our lives. Sometimes our brains can decide it is a good time to deal with other big things at the same time.

Responding to a disclosure of previous trauma

Mandy tells us that her father had alcohol issues, and she has unexpectedly been thinking about her childhood. We may wonder if this has been triggered by the fact that an older man, smelling of alcohol, both traumatised her and damaged her car and then behaved uncaringly. In this setting, we respond with a question based on the present and focusing on current "feelings, thoughts and doing",

> *Sharing now that your father had alcohol problems throughout your childhood, how does that feel?*

Mandy tells us she used to feel helpless and scared then, as she does now. We hear a change in her voice, it becomes quieter and more high-pitched, more child-like. She sounds vulnerable. We notice that we want to tell her, "Everything will be OK" or act in other ways as a nurturing parent because this seems the compassionate thing to do. We may adjust our tone and body language to communicate warmth and empathy, but ask a question whose content keeps us in an adult ego state,

> *When you have times like this, when you feel helpless and scared, what do you do to cope?*

> *How do you comfort that part of you that still feels like a scared, helpless child?*

> *If Mandy, age 7, was here now feeling helpless, what would help her?*

Self-compassion is about giving ourselves the same kindness we would give a friend. Often, we feel that "We should get on with it". Sometimes, bringing the person's younger self into the room allows people to be kind to themselves in ways they feel unable to be with their adult self.

Mandy tells us that her younger self would have loved a hug. We problem-solve with her about possible ways to try to create this sensation now – perhaps wrapping her arms around herself or covering up with a weighted blanket.

If we decided to use a metaphor, we may say,

> *It is like a radio; an unwelcome track keeps coming on and we can't stop that. But we can turn down the volume, open the window and feel the air on our face and tell ourselves: you **can** get through – it will pass.*

In our response, we have uncovered and discussed a manageable amount of information and refrained from going further into the past.

What if Mandy wants to share her difficult childhood experiences now?

Retelling should be done only when someone is able to revisit the traumatic experience without being in a traumatic state – otherwise, it may do more harm than good. Initial conversations often focus on helping someone stay "present" using breathing, anchors and body movement. An experience should not be relived without these tools. Also, remember that many people get frustrated with health services when they have to repeatedly retell their story. Ensuring people talk to the right person the first time can be a good aim,

> *Do you think you might want to talk more about these events now or at some point? We could talk about who would be best to be in that conversation with you.*

> *I can listen confidentially. The only time I would talk to you about us breaking that confidentiality would be if it seemed likely there could be harm to you or someone else. Others who could help would perhaps be a therapist who could work with you. If you talked to me, we might feel that a therapist would be more appropriate. That could mean you need to talk through what happened more than once. Repetition might be helpful or unhelpful.*

> *There are also ways of getting support and fully recovering without ever reliving what you went through, if you don't want to. Other options include an eye movement tool called eye movement desensitisation and reprogramming (EMDR) or trauma-focused CBT.*

After a difficult conversation like this, we need to ensure that Mandy has the fit note she requested, a follow-up appointment and a robust safety net.

Learning point – ego states

Ego states are defined in transactional analysis. There are three states: the parent, adult and child states. In general, we will have the most comfortable and useful conversations when both people talking are in their adult ego state.

(Continued)

We may identify that we have been acting as an overly disciplinary parent, directing a patient to take medication without involving them. Or perhaps we retreated into an apologetic, repentant child state, repeatedly saying sorry for not having the answer to the cause of a symptom.

Transactional analysis tells us that if both people accept and engage in "complementary" states (parent:child), then these can endure over many conversations. For example, a health professional who falls into the role of the nurturing but over-bearing parent might say,

> You mustn't think about that. It will upset you. I am going to sort things out for you.

... and the patient may accept being the helpless child. They may say or non-verbally communicate, *I am helpless and need you to make decisions for me and look after me.* This dynamic may feel satisfactory to both people until the situation changes: the health professional needs the person to make a decision or the patient now wants autonomy over their health care.

What can we do?

If one person notices, they can choose to return to an adult state. An adult still shows empathy and care and partnership but does this as between adults,

> I can hear things are difficult and you have found some ways to cope. What, for you, would be a positive step for us to take next?

With the healthcare professional in an adult state and the patient still in a "child" state, there is now a "crossed state", which is unstable. Either we would need to return to a parent state – nurturing or perhaps disciplining,

> It really is time you made a decision.

... or the patient will need to move to an adult state.

Example 2 – suicide attempt/A&E discharge

The idea of someone talking about ending their life can feel threatening. We worry because of our professional responsibility and might find it hard to approach this discussion non-judgementally. This makes it hard to listen with curiosity and understand the pros and cons and alternative solutions.

We need to be able to listen carefully because we might then be able to find a number of otherwise unimagined solutions. If we can get alongside someone, they may feel there is someone on their team and they are less alone.

Paradoxically, exploring suicidal thinking and actions with curiosity may well reduce the risk of this happening.

Tools

- ABC.
- Shrink it.

Patient	Imani McFarlane, 20 years, female.
PMH	A&E note: overdose paracetamol, 10 tablets.
	Marks from cutting noted on arms.
	Reviewed by psychiatrist on-call – discharged home.
	GP to follow up please.
Social history	Lives with parents.
Behaviour	Very quiet, looking tense and angry.
Opening statement	*They told me to come. It was another bad decision.*

Imani looks down, she's waiting for us to start.

What do you say now?

We try,

> *I was just looking at your notes from the hospital. You have had a really big 24 hours. How are you feeling today?*

Imani tells us that she is feeling OK today. She was told to come in for "follow-up" after the overdose.

She frequently argues with her dad. He is very traditional and disagrees with her life plans. He wants her to be *like you* – work in healthcare or something similar. He doesn't understand that she is an adult, living her own life. He says it is his house and his rules.

Living with a friend didn't work out, so she has been home for the last three months and it feels like a pressure cooker. She has also recently argued with her boyfriend; he had been supportive but now she feels he doesn't understand her either. She thinks she may need to move to a new place and start afresh.

There is quite a lot of information here. We structure and add to it using ABC.

Responding to suicidal thinking – ABC

Particularly when someone has judged themselves, as Imani has – *another bad decision* – we can normalise the thinking and talk through what was happening "before", "during her actions" and "now". We use the psychological tool ABC to help structure the conversation,

Antecedents – "before"

> *Before you took the paracetamol, what else were you thinking or feeling and what did you do? Was there a particular trigger that finally tipped you to take the paracetamol?*

Behaviour – "actions"

> *When you were deciding to take the paracetamol, did you consider any other actions? At that moment, did you have a particular outcome that you wanted?*

Consequences – "next and now"

> *What happened straight after you took the paracetamol? What were you thinking and feeling? What did you do? How do you feel now, looking back? What would you say are the pros and cons of this action?*

These questions help us stay non-judgemental, listening and curious.

Imani was alone in her room, staying away from arguments downstairs. She was relaxing, drinking vodka and started to feel alone, with no one to talk to. She had thought she would be with her boyfriend, Freddie, forever, and now she feels really disconnected from him. Then she started thinking about still living at home with a disapproving dad and no career plan.

Suddenly, she decided she wanted to go to sleep to stop all the thoughts. She took the paracetamol but collapsed on the bathroom floor. Her mum heard, came straight up and took her to A&E. She feels embarrassed now, *another bad decision*. She doesn't currently have any thoughts of ending her life or self-harming again.

We reflect back,

A *Last night your thoughts were running in a lot of directions – family, relationships, career. Having all those thoughts going round and round is exhausting. I can understand you wanting a way of "escaping" from that non-stop thinking.*

B *It was quite a sudden decision – you went to the bathroom thinking of taking medication to help you sleep, then took the paracetamol.*

C *In a way, it did work: you were lonely, but then your mum was with you. However, you had to go to hospital and felt embarrassed and that you had made a bad decision.*

We have used ABC to help increase our, and Imani's, understanding of the situation, and this has started to yield potential ideas to use in a plan going forward.

Agree – "shrink it" direction

Imani has told us about an overwhelming number of issues, so "shrink it" is a good tool. We can think about using this whenever we, or the person we are talking to, appear to feel overwhelmed. If someone's safety is at risk, then "shrink the time, grow the team" is a go-to strategy.

"Shrinking" means we can consider just one decision or situation – consciously parking other life decisions to ensure a safety plan. First, we decide to get consent for this approach,

There is a lot going on for you – thinking about your career options, relationships and even where to live. That can feel overwhelming. How would you feel if we focus on one step for now and come up with a plan to keep you safe for today and this week?

When you are feeling safe and we have some foundations in place, it can feel easier to make other decisions. Shall we focus on a safety plan today?

Safety planning

What are other things you have tried in the past that have helped you get some relief from all the intense thinking?

This is a coping question. We can look for times in the past when she has used alternative ways of coping to deal with different types of stress. Or we might ask about things her friends use or anything she has thought about trying to help her manage the current stress.

Imani talks about cutting, which gives relief. She started when younger but, in the last few months, has used this now and again and it lets out stress. For other stresses, like exams or arguments with friends, normally she would have phoned her boyfriend or other close friends. We ask about other ways of relieving stress that she has thought of or might try.

She was in a band at school – music is helpful but has caused arguments with her dad, so maybe moving out would help. We bring things back on track – away from a different decision about moving out of home – to the agreed "shrink it" safety plan,

There are lots of different decisions, like moving out. Coming back to ideas to help your brain get a break from all the thinking, I'm hearing a few options – talking to someone close to you, playing music, cutting.

If we imagined you were back in your room with the thoughts getting bigger, what could you try to "turn the volume of thoughts down"?

We decide on a plan – listen to music through headphones. Writing poems is another option. Imani starts to wonder about career options, including poetry, and we again check the agreement to continue to use the "shrink it" approach,

Your brain is thinking about your options for your career and other areas of life. We could easily get sucked in and talk about this now – but I've heard that these thoughts circling and growing can be a problem, so it's worth us talking instead about how to cope with that.

Is it OK for us to continue talking about ways to deal with the thoughts, so you have a plan, if the same things happened again?

How do I get consent to grow the team, when someone is reluctant?

Imani has mentioned good friends and her boyfriend, and we ask,

If someone was going to be involved now, today, who would you find most supportive?

After discussion, she decides on her mum. Keeping a trauma-informed approach can be more challenging when we really want to "grow the team" as part of a safety plan, but also want to avoid a sense of coercion. Listening and understanding the reason for someone's reluctance to involve others is important. It may be helpful if we can agree:

- What information is shared, e.g. only talking about future planning, not past events.

- Identifying if there are certain words or phrases that will not be used.

- Ensuring the person knows this does not change normal confidentiality or entitles this person to automatically be able to access any information without their consent.

- Having the flexibility to change the person involved and that this decision can have an end date/review date.

We discuss the plan with Imani,

If you did find yourself in a similar situation to yesterday and you started to feel overwhelmed, the plan is to try listening to music or working on your poetry. If the thoughts are still bothering you, who could you talk to?

Imani confirms her mum. Note that we used an open question and partnering language when developing the safety plan, jointly deciding who to involve. The more worried we are, perhaps with a younger patient or if the situation is likely to recur, the more we would wish to involve the "backup" team member before ending the conversation. Imani agrees we can phone her mum during the consultation and together they agree that if Imani texts from upstairs or comes down wanting backup, they will either watch Netflix together or visit her grandmother.

Alcohol use increases spontaneous risky behaviour so we should discuss this as part of a safety plan – for her to reduce or ideally stop alcohol. If she does drink, she should not do so alone.

We end the conversation by discussing access to means. Imani and her mum agree that her mum will remove any paracetamol and other medications from the house and any sharp objects from the bathroom.

Safety net

After completing a clinical assessment, perhaps using a screening tool and considering the overall clinical picture, we can decide whether we need specialist services to keep Imani safe. Finally, we include a backup option and a way to contact professional services any time of the day or night – a 24/7 helpline. We arrange a follow-up to review the plan soon and may include another "team" member – in this case, involve Imani's mum to also attend the next appointment.

Understanding normal reactions to trauma

Many people experience traumatic events but few experience suicidal ideation or attempt suicide, though there is an association. The closest association is when the trauma is inter-personal: between people who may know each other or may never have met before. The trauma could be physical, sexual or emotional.

In our conversation, we may have spotted a "significant statement" (see Chapter 8). We decide to pick up her comment about alcohol and use a trauma-informed consent-based approach to ask,

> You mentioned last time that nothing good ever happens when you drink alcohol. I wonder if, while drinking alcohol, something happened that you didn't want. If so, perhaps it is something you might want support with now or in the future – from myself and the team here, or us working out who else could help.

A few months ago, at a party at her boyfriend's friend's house, Imani was returning from the toilet when one of his friends "came on to her". This was unwelcome and she couldn't understand why she didn't push him off, but she couldn't, and she knew she wasn't drunk. Her boyfriend didn't believe her, and they argued.

We explain,

You might have heard of fight or flight reaction when we are in a danger-ous situation, and the survival part of the brain takes over. We can "fight", defending ourselves, like you expected, or "flight" — run away. But other normal reactions include "freeze", where we can't think or move and "flop", where we disengage from our body and become almost unresponsive. It sounds like you experienced more of a "freeze/flop" than the "fight/flight" that you might have expected. These are all normal ways to respond to the situation you were in.

Imani finds this helpful. She thinks support would be good, particularly when you explain that this doesn't have to involve her disclosing any more details than she wants to. Together you decide this could be the next step. Once this foundation is in place, it could help make the other decisions in her life easier.

Fight, flight, freeze, flop, fawn

The final normal "fight/flight" response is "fawn". Wanting to please and going along with what others want, which may involve feeling disconnected from your body.

General conversational tool – shrink it

We use "shrink it" when things feel overwhelming for either or both peo-ple in a conversation. There may be an overwhelming number of issues, information or decisions. "Shrink it" means we can focus on one priority issue and consciously park the rest,

There is a lot going on and it might even feel a bit overwhelming. Can we focus on a plan for the next 24 hours (or week)?

We can then consider a small step for this smaller amount of time.

Data gathering

While we usually think of "shrink it" in our clinical management to plan next steps, we can use it for data gathering. "Shrink it" can help us focus. Where we are unclear about the story we have been told, we may ask,

(Continued)

To help me understand more about how feeling like this is affecting you, please can you talk me through your day today?

Safety

When we consider safety, we think about how to "shrink the time, grow the team." The more concern we have, the more people we want involved, including other professionals, and the sooner we want their assessment.

Many acute mental health teams use a "shrink it" approach for safety, with regular contact such as daily phone calls and face-to-face reviews. In the same way, in primary care, we can arrange a follow-up soon, and we may include other "team" members such as relatives or other members of our primary care team to assist with more regular contact.

Example 3 – overwhelming emotion, anger

Anger can be due to previous trauma affecting someone's ability to manage emotions. Sometimes, it follows a previous negative healthcare experience. If we are not sure, it may be worth using a trauma-informed approach. We may well think,

But I really don't want to have a conversation with someone who is angry.

This is normal and we may consciously or subconsciously try to end these conversations quickly. It can be particularly challenging to remain curious and non-judgemental. However, if we decide to practise staying in these conversations, we may develop our skills and better help those who have experienced trauma.

Why does this person seem angry with me, what have I done?

Showing anger could be a useful strategy for someone because,

My needs are more likely to be met and more quickly.

I often interact like this, I hardly realise how I come across.

Anger can intimidate others – this helps me feel safe after previous harm.

Perhaps I am actually scared but have learnt that showing anger is acceptable whereas fear is not.

Tools

- What balances that?
- Image or metaphor – the storm.

Patient	Anthony Evans, 43 years, male.
PMH	Fractured metacarpals, right hand.
Social history	Divorced, three children.
	Now in a new relationship.
Behaviour	Tense and flushed. Hands clenched.
Expectations	Referral to psychiatry – suggested by his new partner who has written "Personality disorder – needs to see a psychiatrist" on a piece of paper.
Opening statement	*I have been coming here all my life and no one has ever told me what was wrong, my girlfriend is the one who has figured it out. So do something!*

What would you say now?

Internally notice and name

Before doing anything, when noticing anger, we can reassure ourselves we are capable of staying and having the conversation. We may internally tell ourselves,

OK. – he is angry. I can cope with anger. I can get through this. There is no rush.

Background

We start by finding out more, using very short phrases to allow the high-energy emotion to come out and frequently reflecting back to check that we have understood. We use phrases like,

Keep going.

Tell me more about how this started.

Talk me through that.

Unbelievable.

To show we have heard and understood, we give this summary in a neutral, factual, non-judgemental way, including a normalising "self" comment and naming the emotion in the room,

You had to phone twice for an appointment and waited for ages on hold. You didn't know what was happening or what the plan was for your own health care.

If I had experienced this, I think I would feel angry. It would be confusing and might make me wonder who I could trust.

Anthony agrees that it has made him angry. If someone has experienced trauma or felt disempowered, they may feel out of control and have a loss of autonomy – that things are being "done to them". Working in a trauma-informed, safe way we may use some of these words: "choice", "options", "your decision",

After these recent experiences, I would understand your reluctance but, if you wish, one option is for us to talk more now. I can see what I can do to get things back on track – to bring you the information you need to make decisions about your health and feel back in control.

Another option is we rebook for a different day or I give you a ring at a different time. It is up to you. What feels right for us to do now?

At this point, most people choose to continue the conversation. Occasionally someone will decide not to work with us today. We may then work in a trauma-informed way and, if needed, help to find someone of the gender/ethnicity/culture that is a better fit.

Anthony decides to continue the conversation. We ask him to tell us a bit more about what led to his girlfriend writing this down and him coming in.

Anthony tells us he gets angry quickly, from nowhere, as if something in him snaps. He thinks his relationship may not be helping and decides to end it, then changes his mind and now is unsure but often thinks about it. We reflect this and discuss what to talk about next,

Whether to continue or end your relationship is a big decision and one you are not sure about. You also experience getting angry quickly. Which of those is affecting your life more at the moment?

Anthony says feeling angry is his biggest problem. We explore the emotion further, starting with some questions that are more factual and might be easier to answer and, if Anthony struggles to answer, using a "zoom-in" "think, feel, do" framework,

When you have been angry, what have you thought about or done?

Can you talk me through a recent time when you felt angry?

Thinking about it now, what do you feel most angry about?

Who do you feel most angry with?

Anthony is unsure at first, but then identifies he feels angry with his ex-partner for limiting his contact with his children and angry with himself for letting this happen. He didn't see his own dad much when he was growing up and he always said he wouldn't be like that.

What balances that?

A problem-solving discussion reveals that he is currently unable to have regular in-person contact with his children. His lawyer is involved and working on his behalf. He has a phone call with his children once a week, after school on Fridays. We reflect and reframe the situation,

Your kids are really important to you and it is very hard not having regular face-to-face contact with them. Your lawyer is looking into this. By having a regular Friday call, it sounds as if you are doing everything you can right now to have as much contact as possible.

When you feel angry and really want to see your kids and can't, maybe that creates more anger because it feels unfair and out of your control. Do you have any different thought that balances this? Something you can think about that gives other feelings that are different from these angry feelings?

Anthony is not sure but agrees it is true that he is doing everything he can. We notice his low self-compassion and try to reframe, aiming to increase this,

You said that sometimes you tell yourself, "I have ended up being exactly like my dad", and beat yourself up with these sorts of thoughts. Do you ever balance this by telling yourself something like, "I am a loving parent and am willing to do everything I can in order to spend time with my kids?"

When someone hears these statements that they have not previously thought about, it can be a profound moment in a conversation and may be followed by a pause or a comment such as *I hadn't thought about it like that* or an affirmative response.

Image or metaphor – the storm

We may leave the next part of the conversation, potentially returning to it later. When we do go ahead, we could ask a question to understand what being angry looks and feels like for Anthony,

Tell me about some recent times you have felt angry.

What would we see if we were watching a film of you being angry?

What have been the biggest or most worrying recent "angry actions"?

Anthony tells us that he and his girlfriend have recently ended up throwing things and have damaged walls and furniture. He can shout or might walk away. We could use the "choose the focus" tool but we decide to use a storm metaphor,

We say,

One way to think about angry feelings is like bad weather. Sometimes, we know there may be a storm ahead, so we can plan ahead and think about what to do when it hits.

Preparing immediately before a storm – "A golden gap"

If a storm is coming, time to prepare is vital. Noticing any early signs of feeling angry is helpful, as it gives you the most time for last-minute preparation. It can be useful to identify these signs – do certain thoughts or body sensations give clues?

What could help balance things at this point? Thinking, *I am a loving parent doing everything I can to have contact with my kids in this current situation*, or a sensory strategy that can quickly communicate with our brains. We might suggest:

- Listening to a podcast.
- A kinaesthetic strategy such as a stress ball.
- Trying some different smells or scents.

Preparing when there is no storm in sight

It can be useful to prepare before we see a storm coming. Having strong foundations in place will put us in the best position to cope with a future storm. These strong foundations are the ways we look after ourselves, such as showing kindness to ourselves during times of stress to support our health.

We ask Anthony what things in his current situation keep him strong and able to cope. If needed, here are some suggestions:

- Planning time alone for 15 minutes after work with no one talking to him.
- Going for a walk before coming home.
- Enough sleep, healthy food.
- Identifying and contacting calm and supportive people with whom he might spend time.

An expert

Even if the house has been hit by lots of storms, it is still our home and may function, but might benefit from a specialist to undertake maintenance,

Sometimes we might think about seeing someone like a therapist. This can be helpful, particularly if there might be past events that are affecting our day-to-day lives in ways we don't want.

Anthony says this is something his girlfriend wants him to do, and he knows he needs to but he is not sure at the moment. We affirm that we can start other work and review this decision. We agree with Anthony that he will try some of the things we have discussed before making a decision about whether a psychiatrist is needed. He may return with his girlfriend for the next appointment.

Top tips – talking about a decision

Big decisions can feel stressful and, when we are stressed, it can be harder to make decisions. This seems to be the case for Anthony in his relationship. Here is a way to talk about decisions.

Confirm the status of the decision and clarify the options

I'm hearing you are still uncertain about what to do, would that be right? Or do you feel you have made this decision?

So, you are uncertain about whether to emigrate – where there might be more options for work – or stay and keep looking for work here?

Use "On the one hand …. On other hand …."

On the one hand, you have connections here, and it's where your current home is, but you have not managed to find work over the last few months. On the other hand, you wonder whether there might be more opportunities if you move.

(Note that this does not seek to be exhaustive, just to reflect back any reasons expressed for each side of a decision.)

Use values

For you, now, what is the most important thing in life? If you look at the decision from this perspective, does it move you towards one option or the other? Are there other things that are also important?

Endorse the option of potentially not making the decision

Does this decision need to be made now? Could the best decision be to focus on your health, let things settle, and come back to this? What would happen if you decided to put this decision on hold?

Find an action to try

With feeling uncertain about this decision, what would be a small step towards testing out one (or both) of the options?

14

Colleagues

Introduction

Working in the health sector can be stressful for many reasons. We are exposed to other people's traumas, we may work long hours and there is the constant pressure to "get it right" and fear of making a mistake. Our employers, colleagues and patients rightly have high expectations. Errors can cause adverse outcomes and be hard to cope with. We may be the face of a struggling system and personally receive the criticism. Nevertheless, healthcare work can feel immensely satisfying and create lifelong career fulfilment.

Unfortunately, having knowledge and understanding of health does not stop health professionals from experiencing the same range of mental and physical health problems as the rest of the population. How do we support ourselves and our colleagues' mental well-being?

In this chapter, we consider how we might talk with our colleagues about issues affecting their mental health, applying the same tools already described in previous chapters. We consider how to support our colleagues while acknowledging that we are not in the role of their health professional and we may need to encourage them to contact their own healthcare team. We will consider:

- General mental health.
- Anxiety.
- Low mood.
- Sleep.
- Errors or complaints.

DOI: 10.1201/9781003409168-17

Talking about general mental health with colleagues

At work, in the coffee room, your colleague says,

No one appreciates us, I think I have had enough.

Others in the room agree. What would you say now?

We know that secondary traumatic stress, compassion fatigue and burnout may affect those who work in health care and may present with symptoms similar to anxiety or depression. They may also co-exist.

Secondary traumatic stress

Secondary trauma means the distress caused by hearing details or seeing the aftermath of a traumatic event experienced by others. Such events could include sexual assault, physical assault, violent injuries or accidents. Secondary trauma may occur after just a single experience.

Working in health care, we are at risk of secondary trauma because we are exposed to trauma through our patients and also, potentially, our colleagues, who may tell us about their own patients' trauma.

Secondary trauma may lead to symptoms similar to those seen in PTSD, such as flashbacks, nightmares and anxiety.

Compassion fatigue

In compassion fatigue, there has usually been prolonged exposure to many traumatic situations. These can include conversations in which we break bad news of a terminal diagnosis, seeing people become increasingly unwell, providing care for those with mental health needs or being threatened while at work.

Burnout

Burnout is a type of work-related stress that may occur when someone has been exposed to excessive and prolonged stress at work. This may include being faced with more tasks than it is possible to complete in the time available.

Any of the above – secondary trauma, compassion fatigue and burnout – will have emotional costs, affecting mental well-being. They may also overlap, causing feelings such as frustration, being overwhelmed, detached or irritable; cynicism or hopelessness. There may be physical symptoms; headache, poor concentration or disturbed sleep. Burnout may lead to exhaustion.

These states put us at risk of a new or worsened anxiety or depression. They may lead to isolation, stopping activities we usually enjoy, use of alcohol or substances, or suicidal thinking.

Understanding the risks and impacts of these conditions may motivate us to have proactive discussions about mental health in the workplace. Further prompts could be new team members or changes in people in a leadership role, recent staff absences or increased workload.

Here are some questions that could be discussed as a group of healthcare colleagues,

As a team, how will we be aware of each other's mental health needs?

How will we recognise if any of us are having a tougher time?

What is one thing we can do individually and as a group to respond to each other's mental health needs?

How can we support ourselves at times when we might be supporting colleagues?

What do we need from the system? How can we put this in place and let everyone know?

What is one thing we could change today to improve the mental health of one (or all) of us?

Talking about anxiety with colleagues

We will next consider how to discuss generalised and specific situational anxiety.

Generalised anxiety

You are in the staff room with a colleague, and they say,

I'm just so worried about everything.

What do you say now?

We want to respond as a colleague, not as a health professional. Various factors may influence how we respond, including:

• The time we have available.
• Our relationship with our colleague.
• Any former relationship we may have had, for example as a supervisor or mentor.

Here are some ways we may respond.

We may ask a question,

Do you think something has triggered this? Or is making it worse?

Is this more at work or out of work?

Are there particular situations at work when this can feel worse? Better?

We may make an authentic positive statement,

I value being in a team where we can talk about this.

Thanks for being open about what's happening to you.

I think it is important that we, as health professionals, can talk about how we can support our own physical and mental health.

For some people, at some times, we may decide to make a relevant self-disclosure,

I have times, too, when my brain does a lot of worrying.

I find if I've had stress at work and not exercised as much as usual, I am more likely to feel anxious.

I don't know how similar it is to what you are feeling, but in the past, I've also had times when I have worried about everything.

We may ask about the role of the work team,

What are the best ways I/we can support you today?

What can I/we keep doing/change so that when you are here at work, you feel as supported as possible?

Is it worth involving anyone formally, your supervisor or HR?

We may ask about their team outside of work: sometimes, whilst remaining in the role of colleague, we may feel able to ask about who is or could be supportive,

Do you have people who are supporting you with this?

Do you need any help to find the right people to support you?

Example

Sometimes, perhaps when we have limited time, we may take a problem-solving approach, "shrink the time" to the rest of today and say,

Can we think of some ways I can support you with this over the rest of today?

Let's make time later today to see how you have found this.

Specific anxiety

I am stressed about this exam, and I don't think I will pass. Maybe it is better if I don't sit it this time.

What do you say now?

How can a supervisor talk with junior colleagues about situational anxiety?

Discussing anxiety using think, feel, do (body and you)

We would start by saying,

We can all feel anxious at times. If we can identify what happens to us when we are anxious, we may be able to find ways to feel calmer and able to be at our best. Let's think of a situation, for example, an exam where something doesn't go as planned or giving a presentation and stumbling over the words.

After setting the scene, or in response to a statement like the one above we might ask,

When someone starts to feel anxious, what might they notice first?

We might give some options,

Commonly we might get a body hint or doom thought. Things in our body might start happening, like sweating or hands shaking. Or we might get doom thoughts like, "Well there's no point now. I have already messed this up". We feel a strong urge to get up and leave.

Which of these would happen to you? Which would be the most obvious? Which would you notice first?

During this discussion we may notice and reflect back non-verbal signs of anxiety or strategies. Maybe someone is fidgeting their hands or tapping their foot and then taking a deep breath.

These questions can work well in a small group where there is camaraderie through realising these experiences are shared, so they become normalised.

In different situations we might notice other ways that we experience anxiety:

A body hint of "fight-flight" with butterflies in the stomach and sweaty palms in exams.

"Avoidance" of presentations.

"Doom thoughts" when expecting colleague feedback or receiving a patient complaint.

Strategies

What do you do when you notice this? What have you tried? How well does that work? Have you tried anything else?

In a group discussion, there is an opportunity to learn from each other's strategies. We might give some options, as follows.

Doing

- Posture – pull your shoulders back, sit tall and smile confidently to yourself.

- Grow – stand up, stretch your arms right up and make yourself as big as you can.
- Breathing – one deep breath, box breathing, focus on a longer exhale.
- Take control – do something to show yourself you are in your body and in control, and then stretch your fingers out as wide as you can or shrug your shoulders up and release them.
- ACT anchor/grounding – push your feet into the ground.
- Connect with surroundings – notice four colours, three sounds and two different textures.

Thinking

- Think about all the praise you have had from patients or colleagues – what thoughts come up for you when reflecting on this positive feedback?
- Think of a reward you can control – a shopping purchase or special dinner after the stressful situation.
- Work through a plan B for the worst case – know there is a safety net. Think, *I will know I tried and can always try again.*
- Perspective – think about what is important in your life – personal health, family health, grateful patients.
- A mantra – *I can do it, I will do the best I can, I know a lot. I can do this, These people deserve to see how many skills I have.*
- Paint the brightest picture – our brain will naturally focus on negatives. In this tool we balance that by thinking about the opposite end of that spectrum: not just a good outcome, but the best possible outcome. What might this be? We think about ourselves performing as the best candidate, impressing everyone, including ourselves. We knew we were good, but **this** good? It is the best performance of our lives and, at the end, there is applause… Anything is possible!

Avoidance

I don't feel well enough to do the presentation today.

If someone has repeatedly rescheduled a potentially stressful event, they may be using avoidance as a strategy for stress or anxiety. We might discuss an activity ladder approach without directly applying it to them,

Presentations can cause anxiety, especially when we have to rebook them. What do you think about a practice run or some other preparation? If you

imagine that doing the presentation is the top rung of a ladder, sometimes people will think about starting with something that is on the very first rung of the ladder?

There may be practical ways we can help to make the situation less stressful, perhaps a smaller audience for a presentation or dividing an assessment into more manageable parts. We might support any existing calming strategies, for example ensuring there is water to drink or having some music playing quietly in the background.

Talking about low mood or depression with colleagues

You receive a text from a colleague,

I can't come in to the meeting today because of my depression. It has been a problem on and off for years but I haven't known how to mention it.

What do you say now?

We want to start a conversation but aren't sure what to say. We would suggest that the worst thing is to say nothing. The tone and content of the discussion will vary depending on whether we are in the role of peer, senior colleague or supervisor.

Here are some options to dip a toe into this conversation.

Authentic statements

I am not sure if I will use the right words, but I want you to know that I appreciate you sharing this. I hope you know that we value you in our team. It can be difficult to balance work with supporting our own mental health. I hope you sharing this means we can try some ways we could support you.

Questions

How have others responded to you telling them this? What was useful about that? What could have been better?

*What is the most helpful thing for **you** that might happen from you sharing this information today?*

Practicalities

Who else is supporting your health?

There may be support options such as counselling and psychology through the workplace, medical insurance or other providers.

How could work be set up so we can still benefit from you?

This might include people to delegate to, the layout of the work day, remote working that continues a connection with the team but removes day-to-day pressures, boundaries around the number of tasks in a day and finish times.

How will we know if taking time off is the best plan?

Time off may reduce stress but also reduce social contact and meaningful activity.

What else can I do to help you feel safe and supported at the moment/this week?

There may be decisions about what might be shared with whom and who would be involved in these conversations with the wider team whilst respecting confidentiality.

Talking about sleep with colleagues

In the kitchen at work, you find your colleague making coffee. They say,

I am on my third coffee. I've hardly slept all week – I just can't get this patient out of my head. I am fine in the day but at night I keep thinking about what I did. Maybe there could have been a better outcome.

What do you say now?

We suspect we are not alone in experiencing end-of-day exhaustion and getting into bed, only to find that our brain decides to run through the day, on repeat, finding worries.

It may well be our patients' health, not our own, that causes us anxiety and insomnia. Thinking about people we have seen and if we made the right decision is a common experience and a frequent cause of "busy brain" stopping us from sleeping.

Here, our role is not to be the health professional, but we may discuss and share strategies for sleep.

Sleep strategy

1 **Recognise** – I am caught in a spiral of worries and rumination.

2 **Ask** – Is this helping? Right now, is thinking about this helping either me or the person I'm thinking about? For example, has it given me:

   • A new diagnosis to consider?

   • A useful test to add?

   ... or am I running through adverse outcomes and mentally beating myself up without anything useful happening?

   • Is this helpful or enjoyable for me?

   • Am I learning something about myself or this topic?

   • Is not much being achieved by it?

   This leads to the final question:

3 **Doing** – Is there anything else I need to do now?

   • Phone an expert colleague.

   • Search guidelines or other resources to see if I should take some different immediate action.

   • Write a note to remind myself to take action tomorrow.

   ... or do I feel that, for the moment, I can justify and stick with the decisions I made?

   Then, if there is nothing useful to do right now:

4 **Acceptance and put aside.**

   • I have done everything I need to do for now.

   • I have thought this through and can think about this again tomorrow.

   • There is nothing else to do now – I can keep these thoughts safely "filed".

   • My brain will keep trying to get me to think about this because it likes to be awake and thinking. I can notice this and then put this thought to one side.

Sleep strategy – treat thought

After deciding if we need to act on any work or non-work issues, we might use a calming technique, either a treat thought or breathing technique. The thought needs to be calm and uninteresting enough to relax us, perhaps a place we want to go or a meal we might prepare.

If this thought becomes too interesting and we notice feeling more awake, we need to return to a calm strategy, such as focusing on breathing.

At this point we might use a metaphor to step back from both the worries and the replacement thoughts.

Sleep strategy – metaphor

We can help our brains observe thoughts rather than getting pulled into them, for example imagining thoughts like leaves on a stream or clouds in the sky. We can notice them move away; perhaps they drift back and we repeat letting them go.

Another image is a supermarket checkout. First, we recognise a thought has pulled us in and scan it through the checkout, and then we imagine sorting it into a labelled paper bag, perhaps "work", "family" or "to-do list". The same thought may return and be rescanned and bagged again. After scanning all the thoughts, if nothing is left, we may even have bags labelled "waiting for thoughts" or "breathing".

Talking about complaints or errors with colleagues

Maybe I am not in the right career. I have hurt someone – the opposite of what I intended. I don't know how I can feel OK about this.

What do you say now?

Although we know that we will all make mistakes and receive complaints, this doesn't make them any easier to deal with. A complaint or error can trigger doom thoughts, meaning we start questioning every decision and may exacerbate low mood, anxiety or depression.

Complaints or errors can significantly affect our emotional and mental well-being and even lead to suicidal thinking. How can we address and support mental health within a conversation around a complaint or error?

We might discuss the stages of adult development, or the brain's negative focus and how to manage it.

Stages of adult development

Many healthcare workers will have core values about relieving suffering, promoting health and empowering others. An error can mean an outcome that is the very opposite of this, which can cause internal conflict and affect our well-being.

It might help us to consider understanding this from a different angle by considering Kegan's stages of adult development.[1] We transition through these with age and can be in-between categories. Few people move into stage 4 or 5.

Stage 1 – Impulsive mind. Seen in childhood.

Stage 2 – Imperial mind. Particularly seen in adolescents, but also adults, with an emphasis on one's own needs and interests. Others' views matter but only **if** there is a direct unwanted consequence,

> *I feel awful. Because of what I did wrong, I may not get selected to go to the conference.*

Stage 3 – Socialised mind. Most adults fall into this category. There is an emphasis on our relationships, and our roles in our family and society. These shape our sense of self. We are very aware of how others perceive us,

> *I feel ashamed and distressed. I have caused harm and everyone knows I made an error.*

Stage 4 – Self-authoring mind. At this stage **we** define who we are rather than letting others, our relationships or roles define us. We own our inner states and values and can question the values of others. We take responsibility for our emotions and explore these, realising we are capable of change,

> *I hold myself to account for this error and harm. I feel ashamed and upset but able to speak about this. I will work with others, guided by my values, to try and address this.*

Stage 5 – Self-transforming mind. At this stage we see ourselves as ever-changing. We are not held prisoner by our own identity. Complexities can be seen, and multiple thoughts and perspectives can be held at once,

> *I accept both that I intended to help and that I caused harm, and I can feel the emotions this has created.*

Conversations around an error or complaint can be an opportunity for us to learn and develop. We may reflect,

> *What emotions do I feel? Shame, guilt, distress, anger?*

> *Is there a consequence I fear?*

> *Do I feel this redefines who I am? In whose eyes?*

> *Can I see myself differently from this experience? Has this experience changed me (my values, who I am) in any way?*

> *Can I hold two contradictory views of myself: that I value relieving suffering, but my action has caused suffering? What does this mean for how I see myself/my identity?*

Brain's negative focus

We know that our brains will focus on the negative. A core task for our brain is to keep us safe, so it is more likely to fulfil this task by finding potential problems. Our brain may interpret an error or complaint as an extreme problem, a "failure", ignoring that everyone is capable of error. It is human nature.

How can we provide a way to balance this? We might check in and ask,

> *Our brains focus on negatives. How easy will it be for you to put this to one side?*

> *What will you try when you notice yourself fixating on this error/complaint?*

Zoom out

> *What motivates you in this role?*

> *What are some of the things that are important to you in life overall?*

Providing balance

Like flipping a coin, we need to be able to balance negative thoughts. What is on the other side of this coin? What thoughts balance this one?

If you did find your brain fixating on the complaint, wanting to define you by this, what thoughts could balance that?

Tell me about positive experiences you have had with patients.

Self-disclosure

I have found it hard to learn to hold two contrasting things, wanting to help but causing harm.

Follow-up

We strongly suggest regularly checking back in with colleagues after an error or complaint and deciding the frequency of this based on the impact on the individual.

Reference

1. Kegan, R. (1982). The Evolving Self: Problem and Process in Human Development. Harvard University Press.

Final thoughts

They are looking away. They do seem stressed. I think I will start with asking a coping question.

Mental health problems can initially appear overwhelming, as they are often intertwined with physical health, social well-being, and wider family and community, but there are many ways we can approach them. We have our traditional tools of listening, prescribing and referring, and these can be enhanced by conversations that focus on very brief interventions. Each conversation is unique and, with more tools, we can be flexible and so have more useful encounters.

Throughout this book, we have described possible ways to approach these very brief interventions in your mental health conversations with examples of questions and phrases. We wish you well in trying these out, adapting them and finding ways to use them authentically in your own consultations.

DOI: 10.1201/9781003409168-18

Glossary of tools and terms

ABC   ABC is an abbreviation for antecedents, behaviour and consequences (including behavioural or emotional response). With an event identified, say a panic attack in the break room, each of the three areas is discussed: triggers and what happened before the event, the actions at the time and what happened afterwards. It is taken from CBT and used in anxiety, depression, substance use disorder and other conditions.

Abuse   In all mental health presentations, consider whether abuse may be a factor that is triggering or perpetuating the health problems. Domestic abuse typically involves a pattern of abusive behaviour towards an intimate partner and may be physical, mental, financial or sexual. Elder abuse can include other areas such as misuse of medication and neglect that occurs within a relationship where there is an expectation of trust.

ACT   Acceptance and commitment therapy is a psychological intervention that is part of the third wave of CBT. The focus is on accepting what we cannot change and putting energy into the things we can change, moving us in a direction that aligns with our values; a committed action that takes place even with us noticing unwanted thoughts or feelings, for example, *I felt anxious but even after noticing this I went to the production to show my support*. Using an anchor may help. See below – 'Anchors'.

Activity ladder   An activity ladder is a way to describe graded exposure. Exposure therapy is a form of CBT. A person is gradually exposed to a feared situation or object, becoming less sensitive and breaking patterns of avoidance. It is used for anxiety, obsessive-compulsive disorder and phobia.

Activity layers   Activity layers are a form of behavioural activation, a skill from CBT. We imagine a cake with layers of activity divided by fillings of time, for example, morning, go for a walk; afternoon, look online for jobs and decide on two to apply for. Behavioural activation can be very important in treating depression.

Add before subtract   Add before subtract is a way of working within a recovery capital framework. (See **Recovery capital**.) Rather than a single focus on reducing or stopping a substance- or alcohol-use, or self-harm strategy, the focus is first on growing recovery capital, whether this is improving housing, finances or physical health or other areas a person has identified as important.

Anchor, ACT   This is a feeling of being present in the moment in your body, for example pressing feet into the ground.

Assertiveness tools   Making our wishes known, expressing our emotions, making requests and saying no are all assertiveness skills that come from behavioural therapy within CBT. This can help social anxiety, depression and unexpressed anger, *I have helped by taking extra shifts in the past. I know we are short-staffed and need to find cover. I am sorry but I have given it careful thought and made a decision that I will not be working any further extra shifts.*

Balancing feelings/what balances that?   This is a tool that seeks to balance a distressing thought or memory with one that reframes the situation and may create feelings of calmness or contentment. This is a form of CBT and aligns with cognitive restructuring. This approach asks people to notice and modify a negative, irrational or faulty way of thinking. Applying this alongside the principle of acceptance, the thought remains but another is added, like two sides of a coin where both exist but we select which side we are looking at.

Breathing   Breathing can become disordered when we experience mental health issues. Without consciously knowing, we may breathe more quickly or shallowly, using our shoulders and accessory breathing muscles. Similarly, breathing pathologies can create anxiety or distress. Breathing can be a useful way to modify how we are feeling but can need careful discussion to be acceptable.

Calm mind, calm body   We use this slogan when discussing sleep. We need to feel that both our mind and body are calm. Strategies can focus on ways to feel safe and relaxed in our mind, e.g. writing down worries before getting into bed, and body, e.g. gentle stretching exercises before bed.

CBT   Cognitive behavioural therapy or CBT appears in guidelines for numerous mental and physical health conditions. It is a talking therapy that builds an understanding of the connections between our feelings, thoughts and behaviours. Modifying one of these changes the others. Ideas such as mindfulness and acceptance have come from later waves in the development of CBT.

CBT, five-part model This five-part model is a way of considering a situation and the thoughts, feelings, physiological changes and behaviour that accompany it. It can be a discussion or completed on paper. A summary of a completed model may be, *When you saw the building, your heart rate picked up, you stood still and thought others were looking at you, which made you embarrassed as well as anxious, you then turned around and went back home.*

Choose the focus Choose the focus is a way of talking about mindfulness. This is an approach that looks at ways to connect with ourselves and/or where we are physically at a point in time. It does not seek to delete, distract or forget other emotions or thoughts that may be present and causing distress, rather the focus grows to include awareness of other things as well as the distressing thought or emotion. It is a way of "zooming out". *I feel helpless* or *I notice the warmth of the room, wiggling my toes in my shoes and the sound of someone cutting their lawn and I notice the feeling of helplessness, alongside a much smaller feeling of hope.*

Coping questions This involves using questions about how someone is coping in order to identify strengths and current strategies. Such questions often need to be asked twice to find out the strategies. *With all of this going on, what are the things you are doing that are helping you to cope? ... Yes, it might seem like you are not coping. What do you think gets you through day-to-day?*

Core beliefs The term "core beliefs" comes from CBT and refers to our most deeply held assumptions about ourselves and the world, e.g. *I am unlovable.* Core beliefs are formed from our past experiences and tend to be very influential in determining what we think, do and feel.

DBT Dialectical behavioural therapy is a form of third-wave CBT. It follows a structured approach and includes four components. These are mindfulness, interpersonal effectiveness, distress tolerance and emotional regulation. It works well for people who feel emotions very intensely. It was first used in personality disorders and interpersonal conflicts. There is also evidence for its use in mood disorder and suicidal ideation and self-harm. It can be useful to know how to refer to DBT.

HOLLA 321 HOLLA 321 is a tool for discussing suicide risk and making a safety plan. Before using this, we may use thoughts, plans and actions (TPA) questions alongside clinical judgement to check if there is already a plan or action that means a specialist team needs to be involved now. With this excluded, these questions are a way to assess how intrusive and distressing thoughts of suicide are and to come up with a plan to manage these in future. The plan uses themes found in many safety plans, including strategies that a person can do without anyone else, ones that involve other people and having a backup person or way to contact a professional at any time, day or night.

ICE This represents the communication skill of ideas, concerns and expectations. *What thoughts have you had about what has been going on? What is your biggest worry? What did you think we might discuss today, as a next step?*

Identifying strengths This involves reflecting and discussing the strengths and skills someone has. *I am hearing that there has been a lot of pain, you have had to keep picking yourself up again and, however exhausted you have felt, you have done that.*

Identify, assign, discuss (detective, judge, reporter) This is typically used to introduce discussing mental health in a physical health consultation. Wearing a detective hat, we might ask about worries caused by the physical pain, then as a judge, we might evaluate whether we think either the physical or the mental health problem is causing most impact; and finally, in the role of a reporter, we discuss.

Image or metaphor Metaphors are widely used in medicine as a tool to aid communication and avoid jargon. Metaphors may be used to help patients understand the psychological and physical aspects of health and how these are related. *It is going to be a journey; we can take the first step today.*

Life raft A topic that someone finds easier to talk about might be commonly used with young people. For example, someone who is finding it hard to speak about their anxiety may be able to discuss family, a hobby or weather and we might use this to build rapport, allow time for the relationship to develop, and then return to talk about mental health.

Magic wand A magic wand question can help with finding someone's values or what is most important to them in life. It is a way of "zooming out". An example would be to ask, *What would things be like today, if we had a magic wand?*

Motivational interviewing (MI) MI is a collaborative, person-centred way to strengthen motivation and capacity for change while recognising the autonomy of the person. It uses open questions, affirmations, reflections and summaries.

Positive reframing Positive reframing involves thinking about a negative or challenging situation or thought in another way. It is a way of applying positive psychology, for example, *It makes me stressed being stuck living at home with my family. Alternatively, it does give me the time and opportunity to not have to do shopping or meal preparation and instead to focus on my online presence.*

Positive psychology   This is the scientific study of human flourishing or what makes life most worth living as individuals and collectively. In conversations, we can be attentive to the expertise and strengths someone has demonstrated, and reflect these back to them. We may discuss things someone is grateful for and be forward-looking.

Pivot or switch   This is a conscious decision to move a consultation in a different direction. We typically use this when moving from a focus on problems or deficits to instead focus on strengths and possible solutions. A pivot or switch could also mean actively moving from discussing past experiences to considering future desired direction and next steps.

Problem-solving   Problem-solving therapy seeks to define a problem and possible solution and to develop a plan to address an issue, for example, *I am too anxious to go to the supermarket; while working on an activity ladder plan, I will try using online shopping and delivery.*

Recovery capital   This is a way of identifying internal and external resources and is used to initiate and sustain recovery, typically from alcohol and substance use disorder. Capital can come from social networks, work or meaningful activity and a person's values.

Safety plan, three steps   This involves asking questions and finding out what possible steps or actions would keep someone safe, if they were troubled by thoughts of suicide or self-harm. This plan may be shared with a person in written form and, with their consent, with their support people. *When these thoughts bother me, what can I do? Who else can I involve? What's my backup plan?*

Self-compassion   Compassion-focused therapy uses ways to train ourselves to increase our compassion and create feelings of safety and contentment. It includes responding to ourselves with kindness, particularly when we fail, suffer or feel inadequate, and recognises that we are not alone in imperfection and that this is part of being human. Increasing self-compassion helps with depression, anxiety and stress.

Sensory strategies   Coping strategies that use smell, sound, taste, touch, sight and perhaps proprioception – experiment to find what works.

Shrink it   Shrink it is a "zoom-in" approach used when there is a feeling of being overwhelmed. Different factors may be "shrunk":

The time period being discussed, *Let's think about how this has impacted you today.*

The number of problems or symptoms, *It sounds like the pain bothers you but it seems to me your mood is having the biggest impact; can we focus on that today?*

Shrink the time, grow the team   A variation of "shrink it" that can be used in the same situations is "shrink the time, grow the team", which is used for safety concerns. This could mean involving specialist services, or it could mean making contact and involving a support person during the conversation. It may mean offering a next-day follow-up or regular telephone check-ins.

Significant statements   Significant statements can be a cue to someone's core beliefs. They will be a problem if they are overly negative and/or seem like a potentially distorted view. It may be a generalisation, *Oh I will never get it right*, or a hard-hitting statement, *They were embarrassed to be seen with me*.

Sleep   Sleep and mental health are intrinsically linked. Poor sleep can be an early sign of worsening mental health. It can be easy to feel helpless and reject sleep strategies, and these can need careful discussion.

Stress behaviours   Stress behaviours are those things we do when under pressure that enable us to realise that we are stressed – e.g. snapping at loved ones, banging the doors, being aloof or drinking alcohol alone. These are useful to identify so that we can increase our strategies, e.g. *I really snapped then; that is not like me, I think I need to go for a walk after work tonight.*

Think, feel, do (body and you)   This is a way of discussing the CBT five-part model and considering the interactions of our thoughts, feelings and actions. It is a way of "zooming in" to a situation or problem. CBT five-part models are commonly used for anxiety and depression.

Treasure hunt   This method is similar to a coping question but looks for a strategy that may have helped in the past and could be restarted. *What did you do when you felt like this last time? What has been different in day-to-day life since you felt like this?*

Tunnel thoughts   These are a cue that there may be anxiety or concerns, discovered by noticing that the same statement is made repeatedly, e.g. *I think it could be cancer*. This thought is in a tunnel and we keep getting drawn towards it. Even when we have objective evidence that something is excluded, the worries persist. Noticing this can allow us to discuss mental health, perhaps using detective/judge/reporter.

Vowels of change   The vowels of change are a mnemonic based on motivational interviewing. They are a way of remembering an approach that expands on "what are the pros and cons" of a strategy. The principal areas included are the person's **a**im of the strategy, how **e**ffective it is, whether their use of this strategy is **i**ncreasing, what alternative (**o**ther) options they also use and any **u**nwanted outcomes from the strategy.

Appendix – the RCGP curriculum for mental health

The Royal College of General Practitioners (RCGP)[1] curriculum lists many common and important conditions for those learning about general practice in the UK. Some of these are ones that we commonly see and would normally be managed within primary care. Others will require specialist input and we need to know what services are available and how to access them. We have included excerpts from the curriculum here and the full curriculum can be accessed online at www.rcgp.org.uk.

Common presentations that would normally be managed in primary care

Here are some examples:

- Anxiety, including generalised anxiety and panic disorders, phobias, obsessive-compulsive disorder, situational anxiety and adjustment reactions.
- Affective disorders, including depression and mania.
- Bereavement reactions.
- Emotions and their relevance in well-being and mental illness.
- Mental health disorders associated with physical health disorders, e.g. psychosis associated with steroid therapy.

- Depression associated with chronic illnesses such as Parkinson's disease or diabetes.
- Cultural and societal aspects of mental health, including work, spiritual and religious beliefs and practices.

Other conditions that may present in primary care and where we may need to involve specialist help

Here are some examples:

- Abuse, including child, sexual, elder, domestic violence and emotional, including non-accidental injury, where you need to know how to contact safeguarding services and be able to do so.
- Addictive and dependent behaviour such as alcohol and substance misuse. Some GPs will be able to manage these patients in primary care but others will involve local services. Remember that addiction and dependent behaviour is more common in those experiencing mental health problems (termed "dual diagnosis") and is often unrecognised.
- Acute mental health problems, including acute psychoses, acute organic reactions, psychological crises and the application of the Mental Health Act.
- Behaviour problems such as attention-deficit/hyperactivity disorder, enuresis, encopresis and school refusal.
- Self-harm, including putting themselves in dangerous situations as well as self-poisoning, cutting and skin picking. Suicidal thought disorders. Men who self-harm have a higher risk of suicide.
- Eating disorders including morbid obesity, anorexia and bulimia nervosa, body dysmorphia and other specified feeding and eating disorders (OSFED).
- Learning difficulties – the range of mental health problems that people with learning difficulties may experience.
- Mental health disorders due to substance misuse.
- Features of major depression such as psychotic and biological symptoms, bipolar disorder, assessment of suicidal risk and detection of masked depression.
- Obsessive-compulsive behaviours.
- Organic reactions – acute and chronic such as delirium with underlying causes such as infection or adverse reactions to drugs.
- Personality disorders including borderline, antisocial and narcissistic.

- Pregnancy-associated disorders such as antenatal, perinatal and postnatal depression, and puerperal psychosis.
- Psychological problems, including psychosocial problems and those associated with particular life stages such as childhood, adolescence and older people.
- Relationship with substance misuse and dependence, including alcohol and drug misuse and other habit disorders such as gambling.
- Severe behavioural disturbance, including psychotic disorders such as schizophrenia, acute paranoia and acute mania.
- Sleep disorders, including insomnia and sleepwalking.
- Trauma including rape trauma syndrome, PTSD and dissociative identity disorder.

Some ways that patients may present to us

There are symptoms and signs of mental health problems that may overlap with distress and/or physical health problems.

Gastrointestinal
- Abdominal symptoms such as bloating, discomfort and altered bowel habit.
- Appetite changes, including secondary amenorrhea.

Cardiovascular
- Awareness of heartbeat, palpitations, bradycardia, chest tightness.

General
- Sleep disturbance, fatigue, feeling tired all the time.
- Biological features of depression.
- Poor concentration.
- Medically unexplained symptoms (MUS).

Emotional symptoms
- Tearfulness.
- Psychomotor retardation or agitation.

Mental health symptoms
- Hallucinations.
- Thought disorders.

Examinations and procedures that are relevant to patients presenting with mental health problems and that primary care practitioners should be competent to undertake include:

- Relevant physical examinations, including cardiovascular and abdominal examinations.
- Exploring both physical and psychological symptoms and family, social and cultural factors in an integrated manner.
- Assessing and managing suicidal ideation and risk, shared development and implementing an immediate safety plan with a suicidal patient.

The Mental Health Act and specialist treatments

- The Mental Health Act and the Mental Capacity Act, including the role of the GP in detaining patients under the Mental Health Act.
- Electroconvulsive therapy indications and side effects.
- Self-help and psychological therapies such as CBT, eye movement desensitisation and reprogramming, counselling, psychotherapy, psychoanalysis, aversion, flooding and desensitisation therapies.

Comprehensive assessment of general health and specific tools

- Screening for metabolic and cardiovascular risk factors in people with severe mental illness, and minimising these risks through appropriate lifestyle advice and management, including helping people change their behaviour.
- Assessment tools for mental health conditions such as screening for depression, anxiety, postnatal depression, dementia, suicide risk assessment and risk of self-harm.
- Monitoring of treatments such as anxiolytics and antipsychotic medication.
- Relevant physical investigations such as blood tests, ECG and relevant neurological investigations.

Service issues – how it works in practice

Within the practice

Think about how to identify people with mental health problems, the use of practice registers and case finding, and improving access to care for these people. As regards prescribing systems, you must make sure that all prescribing is safe and appropriate, including monitoring and repeat prescribing. You should consider the following:

- The prevalence of mental health conditions and needs amongst your own practice population.
- The difference between depression and emotional distress and avoiding medicalising distress.
- Practice registers for specific mental health conditions and recording the required data.
- The effect of practice systems on continuity of care, e.g. appointment systems that prioritise access may reduce patient continuity.
- Increasing equity of access to primary care and mental health services including potential increased access issues for those who are vulnerable or have different cultural backgrounds.
- The role of case-finding in identifying people at risk of developing mental health conditions, e.g. those with long-term physical illnesses, using effective and reliable instruments where they are available.
- Safe prescribing, including duration of prescriptions, drug interactions and side effects, required monitoring, consequences of overdose, and prescribing in children, pregnant women and the elderly.
- The importance of concordance in mental health care. Supporting patients in making choices about which treatment options may work best for themselves. The ability to choose improves the likely effectiveness of the intervention.

Other services – out-of-hours and community-based treatments

These will vary from place to place, so know what is available locally in your area.

- Urgent care services including emergency departments, liaison psychiatry, crisis services such as "recovery" or "crisis" cafes, and telephone support.
- Voluntary and community services and charities that promote mental health and well-being.
- The range of psychological therapies available including cognitive behavioural therapies, mindfulness, counselling, psychodynamic, psychosexual and family therapy.

Particular groups – children and veterans

- Supporting children in difficulty, and accessing support and advice from specialist Child and Adolescent Mental Health Services (CAMHS) and CAMHS workers in primary care.
- The needs of and services for veterans including the psychological effects of trauma and war (e.g. PTSD).

Additional important content for you to know

- Balancing confidentiality with safeguarding – including liaising with family and carers.
- Models that create an artificial separation between mind and body – these may be particularly useful in understanding psychosomatic complaints, psychological consequences of physical illness and medically unexplained symptoms.
- Social circumstances – how poverty, debt, inequalities and upbringing may affect mental illness; effective management of these social circumstances to aid recovery.
- Work – evidence for the positive relationship between work and mental health, and the association between unemployment and declining mental health.
- Disability and social exclusion – how mental health problems may contribute.
- Long-term health problems – may be associated with depression and anxiety and contribute to increased morbidity and mortality.
- Stigma – the "label" of a mental health problem and how this may be associated with discrimination and isolation.
- Cultural dimensions – sensitivity and awareness that, for example, a psychological intervention may not be acceptable to some people who have alternative explanations for, and understandings of, their symptoms.
- Preventing mental ill health through the well-being agenda, mental health promotion and psychosocial interventions.

Reference

1. The RCGP 2020 Curriculum for Mental Health. (2020). https://www.rcgp.org.uk/mrcgp-exams/gp-curriculum/clinical-topic-guides#mental

Index

Note: page numbers in *italics* refer to figures.

Printed in the United States
by Baker & Taylor Publisher Services